Leonardo Melo

Healthy mouth, healthy wallet

Oral Health on a Budget

Copyright © 2024 by Leonardo Melo

All rights reserved. No part of this publication may be reproduced, stored or transmitted in any form or by any means, electronic, mechanical, photocopying, recording, scanning, or otherwise without written permission from the publisher. It is illegal to copy this book, post it to a website, or distribute it by any other means without permission.

First edition

This book was professionally typeset on Reedsy
Find out more at reedsy.com

Contents

1. Healthy mouth, healthy wallet: Oral Health on a Budget 1
2. The High Cost of Dental Care and Its Impact on Your Wallet 2
3. Fundamentals of Oral Health 5
4. Oral Anatomy 11
5. Common oral health issues and their financial implications 18
6. Dental Treatments: Understanding Your Options and Making Informed Decisions 30
7. Oral Health for Different Life Stages 47
8. Oral Health Myths and Facts 56
9. Oral Health on a budget 60
10. Mastering the Basics: Essential Oral Hygiene Practices 69
11. The Importance of Oral Health 82
12. Nutrition for a Healthy Mouth 85
13. How to set up my preventive care strategy? 112
14. Investing in your oral health, investing in your future 116
About the Autor 119

    1.

    2.

    3.

    4.

    5.

    6.

    7.

    8.

    9.

    10.

    11.

    12.

    13.

    14.

1

Healthy mouth, healthy wallet: Oral Health on a Budget

Good oral health is not just about having a bright, beautiful smile - it's also intrinsically linked to your overall financial well-being. This book explores the connection between oral health and personal finances, providing you with the knowledge and strategies to maintain a healthy mouth and save money on costly dental treatments. From understanding the high costs of dental care to implementing effective preventive measures, this comprehensive guide will empower you with knowledge to understand some of the most common diseases and how to prevent them, this is how you can take control of your oral health and your wallet.

2

The High Cost of Dental Care and Its Impact on Your Wallet

Welcome to your practical and comprehensive guide to saving money while taking care of your oral health. Here, you will discover all the details of the most common oral health issues, their treatment and how to prevent dental problems, avoiding frequent visits to the dentist, and, best of all, save a considerable amount in the process. I am passionate about oral health and committed to providing clear, engaging, and practical information to help you achieve healthy smiles and lower your Dental care anual cost.

When it comes to dental procedures, costs can vary significantly depending on various factors, including the type of procedure needed, the complexity of the case, and the geographical location. However, there are certain times when dental procedures tend to become more expensive. Here are some examples:

Dental Emergencies	Complexity of the Case	Cosmetic Procedures
Procedures performed in emergency situations, such as treatment for acute tooth pain, dental fractures, or oral trauma, often require immediate attention and may result in higher costs, especially if they are outside of regular business hours.	Complex dental cases that require extensive procedures, such as jaw reconstruction surgeries, prolonged orthodontic treatment, or dental implants in multiple areas, can result in substantial costs due to the nature of the work involved.	Cosmetic dental procedures, such as teeth whitening, porcelain veneers, or dental implants, are typically optional and not covered by standard dental insurance plans. Therefore, these procedures tend to be more expensive.

It is important to understand that prevention is key to avoiding expensive dental procedures. Maintaining good oral hygiene, scheduling regular check-ups with your dentist, and treating dental problems as soon as they arise can help prevent the high costs associated with complex dental procedures.

The Cost of Dental Care

Dental care can be a costly expense that many people struggle to afford. From routine cleanings and fillings to more complex procedures like root canals and crowns, the high cost of dental care can take a significant toll on your wallet.

According to a study conducted by the American Dental Association, the average cost of a routine dental check-up and cleaning can range from $100 to $200, depending on where you live and the specific services you require. More extensive procedures, such as fillings, crowns, and root canals, can cost hundreds or even thousands of dollars out of pocket, especially if you do not have dental insurance.

The high cost of dental care can have a major impact on your overall financial health. Many people are forced to delay or skip necessary dental treatments due to the expense, which can lead to more serious oral health issues down the road. Untreated dental problems can result in pain, infection, and even tooth loss, all of which can be more costly to treat in the long run.

For those without dental insurance, paying for dental care can be particularly challenging. Many employer-sponsored health insurance plans do not include dental coverage, leaving individuals to foot the bill for their dental expenses. Even for those with dental insurance, coverage can be limited, with high deductibles, copayments, and annual maximums that may not fully cover the cost of necessary treatments.

To help mitigate the high cost of dental care, it is important to prioritize preventive oral health care, such as regular dental check-ups and cleanings, to catch any issues early before they become more serious and expensive to treat. Additionally, exploring alternative payment options, such as dental savings plans or financing options offered by dental offices, can help make dental care more affordable.

Ultimately, investing in your oral health is essential for your overall well-being, but the high cost of dental care can make it a financial burden for many. By being proactive about your oral health and exploring all available options for paying for dental care, you can help protect your wallet while maintaining a healthy smile.

Saving Money on Dental Care

For people who are looking to save money on their dental care, it's important to understand the potential financial implications of neglecting your oral health. When it comes to oral health, prevention is the most important rule. Regular dental check-ups and cleanings can help prevent more serious and costly issues down the road.

By investing in preventive care, you can catch problems early on and avoid the need for expensive treatments later. Additionally, practicing good oral hygiene at home, such as brushing and flossing regularly, can help reduce the risk of developing not only cavities and gum disease, but can prevent chronic diseases which can also save you money in the long run.

Here some tips if you want to decrease the impact of the high cost treatment:

1. Practice good oral hygiene: Brushing and flossing regularly can help prevent dental issues that may lead to costly treatments. This simple habit can help you avoid the need for expensive dental procedures in the future.
2. Visit the dentist regularly: Regular dental check-ups can help catch any potential issues early on, preventing them from becoming more serious and costly to treat. Prevention is key to reducing the overall cost of dental care.
3. Look into dental insurance or discount plans: Dental insurance can help offset the cost of dental care, making it more affordable for you and your family. Alternatively, discount plans can provide savings on dental services without the need for traditional insurance.
4. Consider alternative payment options: Many dental offices offer payment plans or financing options to help make dental care more affordable. Talk to your dentist about payment options that may work for your budget.
5. Seek out community resources: Some communities offer low-cost or free dental clinics for those in need. Look into local resources that may provide affordable dental care options for you and your family.

3

Fundamentals of Oral Health

Understanding Oral Anatomy and Function

To learn about oral health, we first need to understand the anatomy of the mouth. Here we are going to explain some of the important structures of the mouth.

The main structures of the mouth are Tooth, Gums, Tongue, Cheeks, Palate, and Lips. There are other parts, but they will not be covered here as they are more specific and less relevant for general knowledge

Functions

Teeth

Chewing and Digestion

The primary function of teeth is chewing, which facilitates digestion. When we chew, we break food into smaller pieces, making it easier to digest. Proper digestion is essential for the efficient absorption of the nutrients needed to keep the body healthy.

Speech and Communication

Teeth are essential for clear and correct speech. They help form specific sounds and articulate words. Dental problems, such as missing or misaligned teeth, can cause speech difficulties, affecting communication and, consequently, social and professional life.

Aesthetics and Self-Esteem

A healthy and beautiful smile significantly contributes to self-esteem and confidence. Well-maintained teeth enhance appearance and influence first impressions, which can be important in social and professional situations. Dental aesthetics are not limited to appearance but also include a positive psychological impact.

Support Function

Teeth also play a structural support role for the face. Tooth loss can lead to changes in facial structure, causing an aged appearance and affecting overall looks.

Protection of Oral Structures

Teeth help protect other oral structures, such as the tongue and gums, during chewing and speaking. Healthy teeth prevent injuries to the tongue and gums, providing a safer and healthier oral environment.

Gums

Structural Support

The gums play a crucial role in the structural support and protection of the teeth. They cover and protect the roots of the teeth, helping to keep them firmly anchored in the alveolar bone. Without healthy gums, teeth can become loose and even fall out. Gums help protect teeth against impacts, acidic substances, and cold substances. People with gum recession often suffer from sensitivity in the affected teeth.

Protection Against Infections

The gums act as a protective barrier, preventing bacteria and other pathogens from entering the bloodstream through the areas around the teeth. Gum health is essential for preventing infections that can lead to periodontal diseases.

Tongue

Role in Digestion

The tongue plays an essential role in digestion. It helps move food within the mouth, positioning it between the teeth for chewing. After chewing, the tongue aids in forming the food bolus and moving it toward the throat to be swallowed. Additionally, the tongue is responsible for the perception of tastes, which stimulates the production of saliva and other digestive enzymes.

Speech and Communication

The tongue is fundamental for the articulation of speech. It works in conjunction with the teeth, lips, and palate to form sounds and words. Precise movements of the tongue are necessary to correctly pronounce a wide variety of sounds, and tongue problems can lead to speech difficulties.

Sense of Taste

The tongue is the primary organ of taste. The taste buds located on the surface of the tongue detect five basic tastes: sweet, salty, sour, bitter, and umami. The ability to perceive different flavors not only makes eating more enjoyable but also helps identify potentially dangerous foods, such as spoiled or poisonous ones.

Protection and Cleaning

The tongue helps in cleaning the mouth. It removes food particles and dead cells from the surface of the teeth and gums, helping to maintain oral hygiene. A healthy tongue can prevent the buildup of bacteria that cause bad breath and oral diseases.

Swallowing Reflex

The tongue plays a crucial role in the swallowing reflex. By pushing the food bolus toward the throat, the tongue initiates the swallowing process, which is an automatic movement necessary for safe and efficient eating

Cheeks

Structural Protection

The cheeks play a crucial role in protecting the internal structures of the mouth. They help safeguard the teeth, gums, tongue, and jawbones from external impacts. The cheeks also help cushion shocks during activities such as chewing, speaking, and even accidental falls or blows.

Role in Chewing

The cheeks are fundamental for efficient chewing of food. They help keep food positioned between the teeth while we chew, preventing pieces of food from escaping the mouth. The cheeks also work in conjunction with the masticatory muscles to move food from side to side, facilitating thorough chewing.

Assistance in Speech

The cheeks, along with the tongue, lips, and teeth, play an important role in articulating sounds. They help shape the oral cavity, allowing the production of clear and distinct sounds. The pressure and movement of the cheeks contribute to the formation of specific words and sounds during speech.

Facial Expression

The cheeks are key components of facial expression. Movements of the cheeks, such as smiling, frowning, or puffing, convey a wide range of emotions and social signals. The appearance and mobility of the cheeks significantly influence non-verbal communication and social interactions.

Saliva Production

The parotid salivary glands, located in the cheeks, are responsible for producing a significant portion of saliva. Saliva is essential for oral health as it helps keep the mouth moist, facilitates chewing and swallowing, and **protects against cavities and oral infections**. The cheeks aid in distributing saliva throughout the mouth during chewing and speaking.

Palate

Structure and Division

The palate is the structure that forms the roof of the mouth and is divided into two main parts: the hard palate and the soft palate. The hard palate is the anterior, bony, and rigid part, while the soft palate is the posterior, muscular, and flexible part.

Function in Chewing and Swallowing

The palate plays a crucial role in chewing and swallowing. During chewing, the hard palate provides a rigid surface against which the tongue can press food, helping to form the food bolus. During swallowing, the soft palate elevates to close off the nasopharynx, preventing food or liquids from entering the nasal passages.

Function in Speech

The palate is essential for speech articulation. The hard palate, in particular, helps form consonant sounds such as "t," "d," "n," and "l." The soft palate, by moving, contributes to the production of sounds like "k" and "g" and also plays a role in sound modulation, influencing the resonance of the voice.

Separation of Oral and Nasal Cavities

The palate separates the oral cavity from the nasal cavity. This separation is vital for functions such as breathing and eating simultaneously. Additionally, the palate helps prevent food and liquids from entering the nasal cavity during chewing and swallowing.

Contribution to Taste

The palate also has taste buds, though fewer in number than those on the tongue. These taste buds contribute to the perception of flavors, complementing the gustatory function of the tongue.

Protection and Immunity

The palate plays a role in immune defense. The palatine tonsils, located near the soft palate, are part of the lymphatic system and help fight infections. Additionally, the palate helps protect the nasal cavity and pharynx from the entry of large particles and pathogens.

Lips

Protection and Sealing

The lips play a crucial role in protecting the internal structures of the mouth. They help seal the mouth, preventing the entry of particles, bacteria, and other pathogens. This sealing function is essential for maintaining the moisture of the oral cavity and preventing excessive dryness that can lead to cracks and infections.

Role in Eating

The lips are fundamental in eating. They help keep food and liquids inside the mouth during chewing and swallowing. Additionally, the lips assist in forming the food bolus by directing food between the teeth and facilitating efficient chewing. In liquid suction, especially in infants, the lips play an essential role.

Function in Speech

The lips are indispensable for speech articulation. They work in conjunction with the tongue, teeth, and palate to produce specific sounds. Precise lip movements are necessary to pronounce bilabial consonants (such as "b" and "p") and labiodental consonants (such as "f" and "v"). The ability to control the lips properly is vital for clear and effective communication.

Facial Expression

The lips are key components in facial expression and non-verbal communication. They help convey a wide range of emotions, such as happiness, sadness, surprise, and anger. Smiles, kisses, pouts, and other lip movements play an important role in social interactions and building interpersonal relationships.

Sensitivity and Touch

The lips are one of the most sensitive parts of the human body, filled with nerve endings that make them highly receptive to touch, temperature, and pain. This sensitivity is important for various functions, from detecting foreign objects in food to appreciating different textures and temperatures of foods.

Function in Breathing

Although primary breathing occurs through the nose, the lips also play a role in breathing, especially when the nose is obstructed. They help regulate airflow during mouth breathing, ensuring that the air is filtered and warmed before entering the lungs.

4

Oral Anatomy

Teeth

The most commonly oral treatments are basically performed on one structures: the teeth. To better understand the types of treatments, let's learn a little about the morphological part of this structures.

Teeth are divided into three main structures: the crown, the neck, and the roots. Here's a breakdown of each structure:

Crown

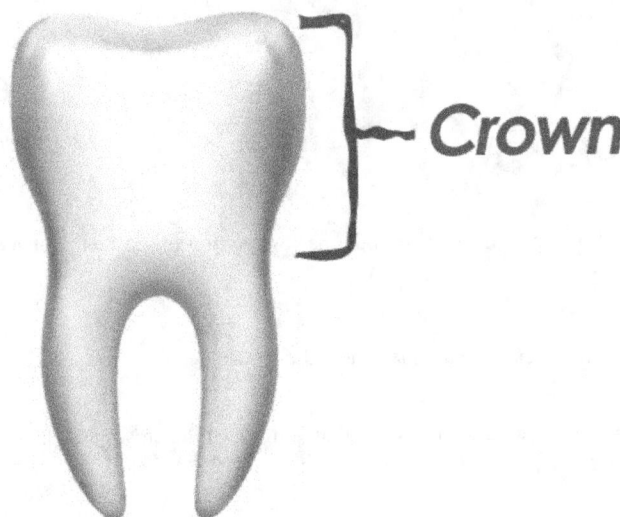

The crown is the visible part of the tooth that protrudes above the gumline.

Location: It is located in the upper portion of the tooth, above the gumline.

Function: The crown is primarily responsible for chewing, tearing, and grinding food.

Composition: Covered by enamel, the hardest substance in the human body, which protects the underlying layers of dentin and pulp.

Neck (Cervix)

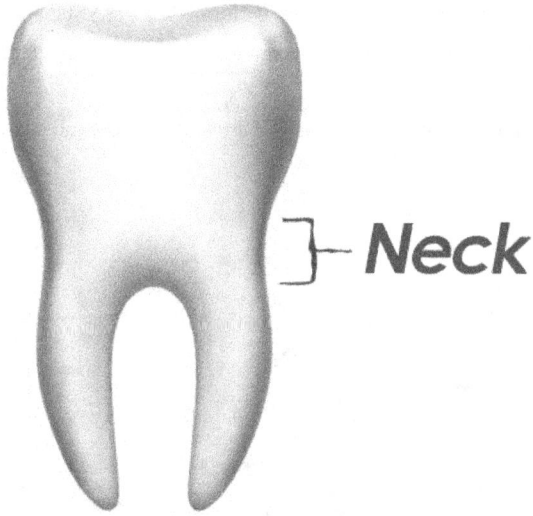

The neck, also known as the cervix, is the narrow portion of the tooth between the crown and the roots.

Location: It is situated at the gumline, where the crown meets the root.

Function: The neck provides a transitional area between the crown and the roots, allowing for flexibility and support.

Composition: Composed of enamel at the crown portion and cementum at the root portion, with dentin underneath.

Roots

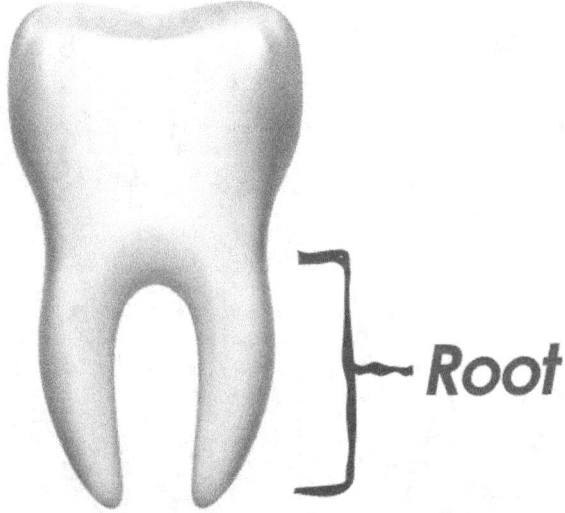

The roots are the portion of the tooth that extends below the gumline and anchors the tooth to the jawbone.

Location: They are located in the lower portion of the tooth, beneath the gumline.

Function: The roots provide stability and support to the tooth, anchoring it firmly in the jawbone.

Composition: Covered by cementum, a thin layer of hard tissue that attaches to the periodontal ligament, which helps secure the tooth in the socket. Inside the roots are pulp canals, which contain blood vessels, nerves, and connective tissue.

This division of teeth into crown, neck, and roots helps to understand the anatomy and function of each part, contributing to overall oral health and function.

Now let's understand about the layers of the teeth:

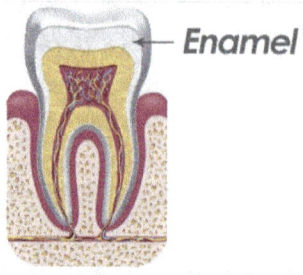

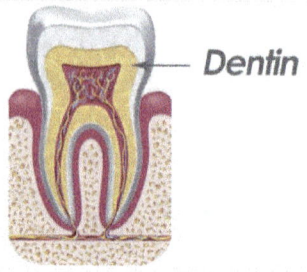

Enamel

The outermost layer of the tooth, enamel is the hardest substance in the human body, providing protection against decay and wear. It is translucent and allows the underlying dentin color to show through

Dentin

Beneath the enamel lies dentin, a hard, yellowish tissue that makes up the bulk of the tooth structure. Dentin is less dense than enamel but still provides support and protection to the inner pulp.

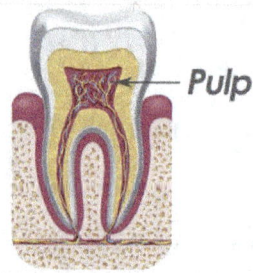

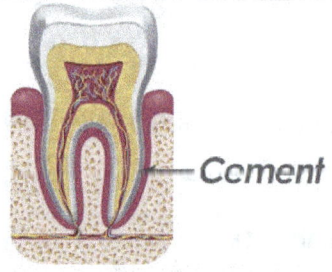

Pulp

The pulp chamber is located at the center of the tooth and contains blood vessels, nerves, and connective tissue. It supplies nutrients to the tooth and responds to stimuli such as temperature and pressure.

Cement

Cement covers the roots of the tooth and helps anchor it to the jawbone through periodontal ligaments. It is similar in composition to bone but is softer and more porous.

Enamel:

　Composition: Enamel is the outermost layer of the tooth and is the hardest substance in the human body. It consists primarily of hydroxyapatite crystals, making it highly resistant to wear and tear.

　Function: Enamel serves as a protective shell, shielding the inner layers of the tooth from decay and damage. It also provides the tooth with its characteristic white appearance and smooth surface, facilitating chewing and speaking.

Dentin:
Composition: Dentin lies beneath the enamel and is slightly softer than enamel. It is composed of microscopic tubules surrounded by a mineralized matrix, giving it both strength and flexibility.
Function: Dentin provides structural support to the tooth and acts as a cushion against external forces. It contains nerve endings, making it sensitive to temperature, pressure, and touch. Dentin also determines the color of the tooth, shining through the translucent enamel.

Pulp:
Composition: The pulp is the innermost layer of the tooth, consisting of soft connective tissue, blood vessels, nerves, and lymphatic vessels.
Function: The pulp serves as the vital center of the tooth, supplying nutrients and oxygen to the surrounding tissues. It also houses the tooth's nerve endings, which transmit sensations such as pain, temperature, and pressure. The pulp plays a crucial role in the formation and repair of dentin throughout life.

Cementum:
Composition: Cementum covers the roots of the tooth and is similar in composition to bone, consisting of mineralized tissue and collagen fibers.
Function: Cementum anchors the tooth securely to the surrounding bone and periodontal ligaments, providing stability and support. It also serves as a protective barrier, shielding the sensitive root surface from external stimuli.

Periodontal Ligament:
Composition: The periodontal ligament is a fibrous connective tissue that surrounds the roots of the tooth and attaches them to the surrounding bone.
Function: The periodontal ligament acts as a shock absorber, cushioning the tooth against forces generated during chewing and biting. It also allows for slight movement of the tooth within its socket, facilitating proper occlusion and alignment.

Alveolar Bone:
Composition: Alveolar bone forms the sockets in the jawbone where the roots of the teeth are embedded.

- **Function:** Alveolar bone provides structural support to the teeth and anchors them firmly in place. It undergoes constant remodeling in response to the forces exerted by chewing and biting, maintaining the integrity of the dental arch.

Gum

Gum anatomy refers to the structure and composition of the gums, also known as the gingiva. The gums are an important part of the oral cavity, serving as a protective barrier for the teeth and supporting structures.

The gums are made up of two main parts: the gingival epithelium and the underlying connective tissue. The gingival epithelium is the outer layer of the gums that is in direct contact with the oral environment, which provides a protective barrier against bacteria and other harmful substances.

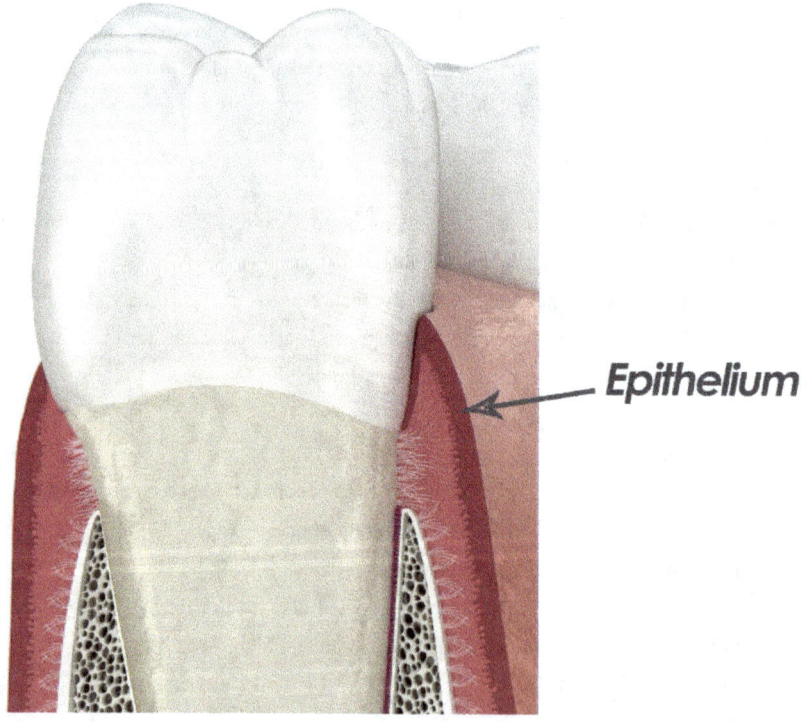

Beneath the gingival epithelium is the connective tissue, which is composed of collagen fibers, blood vessels, and immune cells. The connective tissue provides support and nourishment to the gums, helping to maintain their health and integrity.

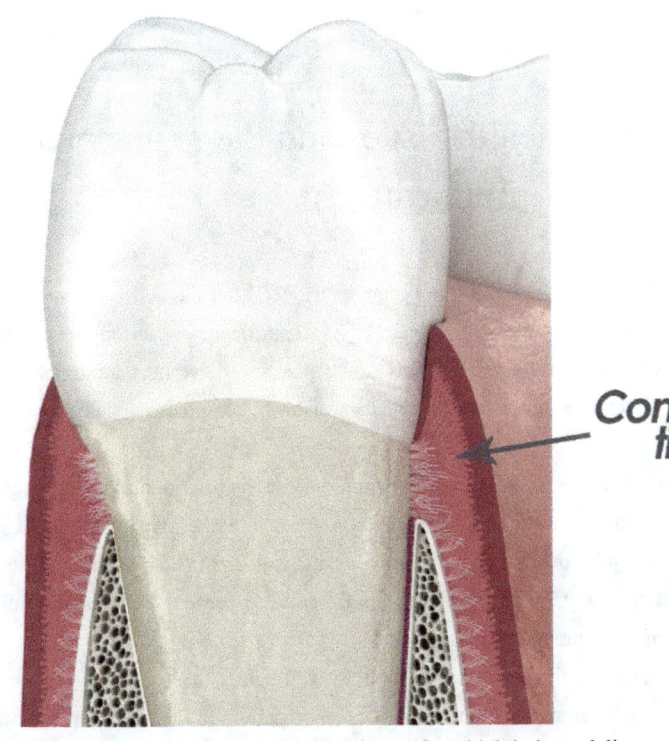

The gums are richly supplied with blood vessels, which help to deliver oxygen and nutrients to the tissues and remove waste products. The blood vessels also play a key role in the immune response, helping to fight off infections and inflammation.

The gums are also home to a diverse population of bacteria, known as the oral microbiota. While some of these bacteria are beneficial and help to maintain oral health, others can cause gum disease if they are allowed to proliferate unchecked.

Proper oral hygiene, including regular brushing and flossing, is essential for maintaining healthy gums. In addition, regular dental check-ups and cleanings can help to prevent gum disease and other oral health issues.

In conclusion, gum anatomy is a complex and important aspect of oral health. Understanding the structure and function of the gums can help individuals take better care of their oral health and prevent problems such as gum disease.

5

Common oral health issues and their financial implications

In the world of healthcare, one aspect that is often overlooked but incredibly important is oral health. The state of our teeth and gums can have a significant impact on our overall well-being, both physically and financially. This subchapter will delve into the importance of oral health and the financial implications that come with it, providing valuable insights for everybody.

Common oral health issues such as cavities, gum disease, and periodontitis can wreak havoc on our wallets if left untreated. The costs associated with these conditions can quickly add up, from regular dental cleanings to more intensive treatments like fillings and root canals. It is crucial to stay on top of your oral health to prevent these issues from escalating and causing even more financial strain.

Maintaining good oral health is crucial for overall well-being. In this chapter, we will explore some of the most common oral health issues and discuss the financial implications of neglecting preventive care. By understanding the potential costs associated with oral health problems, you can make informed decisions about how to prioritize your budget for dental care.

Gum disease and periodontitis treatment costs can be particularly steep, as they often require multiple visits to the dentist and specialized care. Ignoring the early warning signs of gum disease can lead to more advanced stages of periodontitis, which can result in costly procedures such as deep cleanings and even surgery. Investing in preventive measures like regular check-ups and proper oral hygiene can help avoid these hefty expenses.

Similarly, dental cavities and fillings can take a toll on your finances if not addressed promptly. The cost of treating cavities can vary depending on the severity of the decay and the type of filling needed. By maintaining good oral hygiene habits and seeking regular dental care, you can prevent cavities from forming and save yourself from the financial burden of extensive dental work.

Root canal procedures are another dental treatment that can come with a hefty price tag. While root canals are often necessary to save a severely infected tooth, the cost of the procedure and any follow-up treatments can add up quickly. It is essential to address tooth decay early on to avoid the need for a root canal and the associated financial implications. Let's start by looking at the implications of gum disease and periodontitis.

Gum Disease

Gum disease, also known as periodontal disease, is a common oral health issue that affects millions of people worldwide. It is caused by the build-up of plaque on the teeth, which can lead to inflammation and infection of the gums.

It can range from mild gingivitis to more severe periodontitis, which can cause irreversible damage to the gums and bone supporting the teeth. Symptoms of gum disease include red, swollen, and bleeding gums, bad breath, and loose teeth. If left untreated, gum disease can lead to tooth loss and other serious health complications.

The financial implications of gum disease and periodontitis treatment costs can be significant. Treatment for gum disease may include professional cleanings, scaling and root planing, antibiotics, and in severe cases, surgery. The costs of these treatments can add up quickly, especially if multiple visits to the dentist are required.

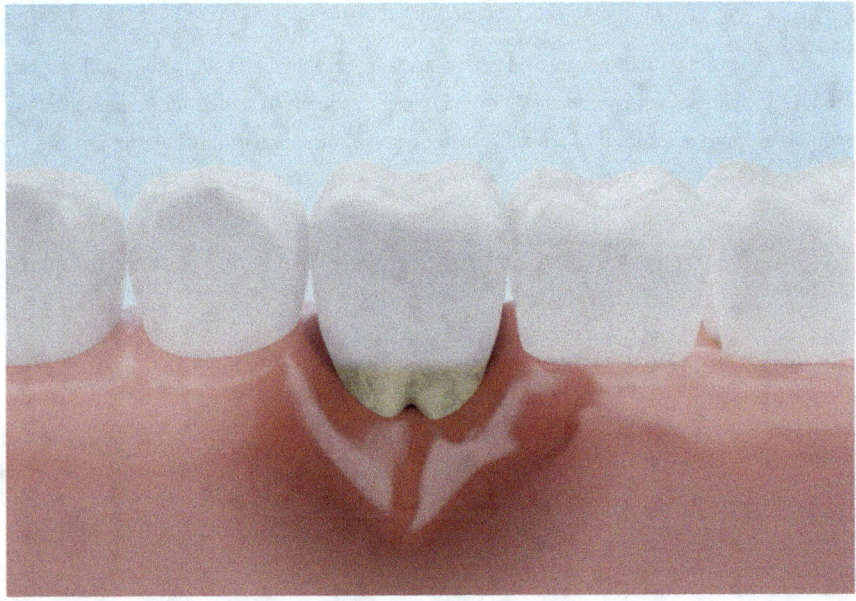

In addition to the direct costs of treating gum disease, there may also be indirect costs associated with the condition. For example, if gum disease leads to tooth loss, the cost of replacing missing teeth with dental implants or other restorative options can be substantial.

Furthermore, ongoing maintenance and preventive care to keep gum disease under control can also impact your finances.

It is important to prioritize your oral health and seek treatment for gum disease as soon as possible to avoid more serious complications and higher costs down the line. By practicing good oral hygiene, including regular brushing, flossing, and dental check-ups, you can help prevent gum disease and maintain a healthy smile without breaking the bank. Remember, investing in your oral health now can save you money and discomfort in the long run.

Tooth Decay

Have you ever wondered what causes those pesky dental cavities that seem to pop up out of nowhere? Understanding the causes of dental cavities is the first step towards maintaining a healthy smile and avoiding costly dental procedures.

Tooth decay, also known as dental caries or cavities, is a common and preventable oral health issue that occurs when bacteria in the mouth produce acids that erode the enamel of the teeth. The formation of tooth decay is a complex process that involves several factors working together.

First, bacteria in the mouth feed on sugars and carbohydrates from the food we eat, producing acids as a byproduct. These acids can gradually dissolve the minerals in the enamel, the hard outer layer of the teeth, leading to the formation of tiny holes or cavities.

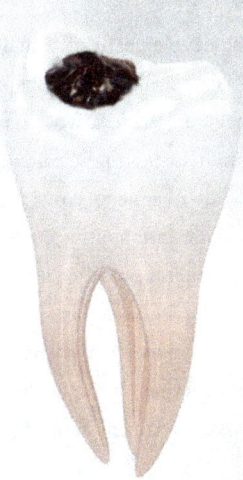

If left untreated, the decay can progress deeper into the tooth, affecting the softer dentin layer underneath the enamel. This can cause sensitivity, pain, and eventually lead to infection or even tooth loss.

Several factors can increase the risk of tooth decay, including poor oral hygiene, a diet high in sugars and carbohydrates, dry mouth, and certain medical conditions that reduce saliva production. Genetics, age, and the presence of certain bacteria in the mouth can also play a role in the development of cavities.

In some cases, dental treatments such as fillings, crowns, or root canals may be necessary to restore and preserve the affected teeth. In severe cases, extraction may be required to prevent the spread of infection to other teeth or the surrounding tissues

One of the primary causes of dental cavities is poor oral hygiene. When we neglect to brush and floss regularly, plaque builds up on our teeth, leading to the formation of cavities. Sugary and acidic foods also play a role in the development of cavities, as they provide the perfect environment for bacteria to thrive and erode tooth enamel. By practicing good oral hygiene and making smart dietary choices, we can significantly reduce our risk of developing cavities and save money on expensive dental treatments in the long run.

Another common cause of dental cavities is dry mouth. Saliva plays a crucial role in protecting our teeth from decay by washing away food particles and neutralizing acids. When we experience chronic dry mouth, either due to medications, medical conditions, or lifestyle factors, our teeth become more vulnerable to cavities. Investing in saliva-stimulating products and staying hydrated can help combat dry mouth and prevent cavities from forming.

Genetics also play a role in the development of dental cavities. Some people are more predisposed to cavities due to factors like tooth shape, enamel strength, and saliva composition. While we can't change our genetics, we can be proactive about our oral health by visiting the dentist regularly for check-ups and cleanings. Catching cavities early on can help prevent more extensive and costly treatments down the line.

Overall, the causes of dental cavities are multifaceted, but by understanding the role of factors like oral hygiene, diet, dry mouth, and genetics, we can take proactive steps to prevent cavities and maintain a healthy smile. By investing in preventive care and making smart lifestyle choices, we can save money on costly dental treatments and enjoy the financial benefits of good oral health. Remember, a healthy smile is not only a reflection of our overall well-being but also a wise investment in our financial health.

Pulpitis

Are you experiencing a toothache that just won't go away? Have you been told by your dentist that you need a root canal treatment? Don't worry, you're not alone! Understanding pulpitis is crucial for maintaining a healthy smile and avoiding further oral health issues.

Pulpitis is an inflammation of the tooth's pulp, can cause severe toothache and lead to root canal treatment or even tooth extraction. Ignoring the symptoms of pulpitis can result in more extensive and expensive dental procedures. It is important to maintain a good oral hygiene and seek professional dental car as soon as possible when experiencing any toothache.

If you're already at the stage where you're experiencing toothache, you're likely dealing with pulpitis. At this stage, prevention no longer has an effect, and you'll need an urgent intervention approach to halt and resolve your problem, and to solve it, you will likely need a root canal treatment.

Root canal treatment, also known as endodontic therapy, is a procedure that is used to treat infected or damaged pulp inside the tooth. During the treatment, the dentist will remove the infected tissue, clean and disinfect the root canal, and then seal it to prevent further infection. While the thought of having a root canal may seem daunting, it is actually a common and relatively painless procedure that can save your tooth and alleviate your pain.

When it comes to the financial implications of root canal procedures, it's important to consider both the upfront costs and the long-term benefits. While root canals may seem expensive at first, they are often more cost-effective in the long run compared to other treatments, such as tooth extraction followed by a dental implant. By saving your natural tooth through a root canal, you can avoid the need for more expensive and invasive procedures down the line.

It's also important to note that many dental insurance plans cover a portion of the cost of root canal treatment, making it more accessible for those who may be worried about the financial burden. Additionally, many dentists offer payment plans or financing options to help make the procedure more affordable for their patients. So don't let the cost of a root canal deter you from seeking the treatment you need to maintain a healthy smile.

In conclusion, understanding root canal treatment is essential for anyone experiencing tooth pain or infection. By learning about the procedure and its financial implications, you can make an informed decision about your oral health care. Remember, a healthy smile is priceless, and investing in your dental health now can save you time, money, and discomfort in the future. So don't delay – schedule a consultation with your dentist today to discuss your options for root canal treatment.

Oral Infection

Oral infections are common conditions that can affect various parts of the mouth, including the teeth, gums, tongue, and throat. These infections can range from mild and localized issues to more severe and systemic conditions. Understanding the causes, symptoms, and treatment options for oral infections is essential for maintaining good oral health

Oral Infection, such as tooth abscesses or infections in the gums, can also pose financial burdens if left untreated. These infection can cause pain, swelling, and even spread to other parts of the body if not addressed promptly. Treatment may involve a root canal, tooth extraction or prescription of antibiotics, all of which can add up in terms of cost. Seeking dental care at the first sign of an oral infection is crucial to prevent further complications and minimize the overall health impact.

Causes of Oral Infections:

Bacteria: The most common cause of oral infections is bacterial overgrowth. Bacteria naturally inhabit the mouth, but certain factors can lead to an imbalance, resulting in infections such as tooth decay (caries) and periodontal disease.

Viral Infections: Viruses such as herpes simplex virus (HSV) can cause oral infections like cold sores or fever blisters. Other viral infections, such as human papillomavirus (HPV), can lead to oral warts or even oral cancer.

Fungal Infections: Fungi like Candida albicans can cause oral thrush, a condition characterized by white patches on the tongue, inner cheeks, and throat.

Poor Oral Hygiene: Neglecting oral hygiene practices such as brushing, flossing, and regular dental check-ups can increase the risk of oral infections by allowing bacteria and other pathogens to thrive in the mouth.

Weakened Immune System: Certain medical conditions or medications that suppress the immune system can make individuals more susceptible to oral infections.

Halitosis

Halitosis, commonly known as bad breath, is a condition characterized by unpleasant odors emanating from the mouth. While occasional bad breath is common and often temporary, chronic halitosis can be a source of embarrassment and may indicate underlying oral health issues or systemic conditions. Bad breath can be caused by various factors such as poor oral hygiene, dental infection or underlying health conditions. Ignoring and not addressing its cause can gave social and professional consequences, as is can negatively impact personal interactions and self-confidence. Seeking professional dental care to diagnose and treat the underlying issue can help alleviate and prevent potential long-term complications. Let's see some of the causes of Halitosis:

Poor Oral Hygiene: The most common cause of bad breath is the buildup of bacteria in the mouth, which can occur due to inadequate brushing, flossing, and tongue cleaning.

Food and Drink: Certain foods and beverages, such as onions, garlic, coffee, and alcohol, can contribute to temporary bad breath due to their strong odors.

Tobacco Use: Smoking and chewing tobacco can lead to chronic bad breath by drying out the mouth and leaving behind foul-smelling compounds.

Dry Mouth: Saliva plays a crucial role in washing away food particles and bacteria in the mouth. Dry mouth, or xerostomia, can occur due to factors such as medications, medical conditions, or mouth breathing, leading to halitosis.

Dental Issues: Dental problems such as gum disease, tooth decay, oral infections, and poorly fitting dental appliances can harbor bacteria and contribute to bad breath.

Systemic Conditions: Certain systemic conditions such as diabetes, liver disease, respiratory infections, and gastrointestinal disorders can manifest as halitosis.

Morning Breath: Reduced saliva flow during sleep can allow bacteria to proliferate, leading to "morning breath" upon waking.

Tooth loss

Tooth loss, a condition that affects millions of people worldwide, is often perceived primarily as a cosmetic issue. However, its implications extend far beyond aesthetics, impacting physical health, psychological well-being, and quality of life. It can significantly impair an individual's ability to chew food properly, leading to dietary restrictions and poor nutrition. People with missing teeth may avoid hard or fibrous foods like fruits, vegetables, and nuts, which are essential sources of vitamins and minerals.

Are you wondering why your dentist is recommending a tooth extraction? There are several reasons why this procedure may be necessary for your oral health. One common reason for tooth extraction is severe damage or decay that cannot be repaired with a filling or crown. In some cases, a tooth may be too damaged to save and must be removed to prevent further infection or pain. Additionally, overcrowding of teeth can also be a reason for extraction, especially in cases where orthodontic treatment is needed to align the teeth properly.

Gum disease and periodontitis can also lead to the need for tooth extraction. If the infection has spread to the bone supporting the teeth, extraction may be necessary to prevent further damage and preserve the health of the surrounding teeth. The cost of treating gum disease and periodontitis can add up quickly, making prevention through regular dental cleanings and check-ups essential to avoid the need for tooth extraction.

In cases where dental cavities have progressed to a point where a filling is no longer a viable option, tooth extraction may be recommended. The cost of treating cavities and fillings can vary depending on the severity of the decay and the type of filling material used. However, the cost of a tooth extraction may be higher than that of a filling, making prevention through good oral hygiene practices crucial to avoid the need for extraction.

After a tooth extraction, there are additional costs to consider for post-surgery care, such as pain medication, follow-up appointments, and potential complications. It is important to follow your dentist's recommendations for post-surgery care to ensure proper healing and prevent infection. By understanding the reasons for tooth extraction and the associated costs, you can make informed decisions about your oral health and budget for any necessary procedures.

The loss of teeth can have a profound impact on an individual's self-esteem and confidence. A full, healthy smile is often associated with attractiveness and social success, and tooth loss can lead to feelings of embarrassment and self-consciousness. This can affect personal and professional interactions, leading to social withdrawal and isolation. Chronic embarrassment or dissatisfaction with one's appearance can contribute to mental health issues such as **depression and anxiety**. Studies have shown that individuals with missing teeth are more likely to experience psychological distress, which can affect overall quality of life. The stigma associated with tooth loss can exacerbate these feelings, making it difficult for affected individuals to seek help.

Poor oral health can also impact your overall health and well-being, leading to systemic conditions like heart disease, diabetes, respiratory infections and even mental health issues. The financial burden of managing these health conditions can be significant, emphasizing the importance of prioritizing oral health as part of your overall healthcare routine. By taking steps to prevent oral health issues, you can potentially reduce your risk of developing costly chronic diseases and save money on healthcare expenses in the long term.

Oral Cancer

Oral cancer encompasses cancers of the lips, tongue, cheeks, floor of the mouth, hard and soft palate, sinuses, and throat. It is a serious condition that can be life-threatening if not diagnosed and treated early. Major risk factors for oral cancer include tobacco use (including smoking and smokeless tobacco), heavy alcohol consumption, human papillomavirus (HPV) infection, excessive sun exposure to the lips, and a diet low in fruits and vegetables.

Diagnosis and Treatment: Diagnosis typically involves a thorough examination by a healthcare professional, which may include a biopsy of the suspicious area, imaging tests such as X-rays, CT scans, MRIs, and PET scans to determine the extent of the cancer.

Treatment depends on the stage and location of the cancer and can include:

- **Surgery**: Removal of the tumor and possibly some surrounding tissue. More extensive surgery may be needed for larger tumors or if the cancer has spread.
- **Radiation Therapy**: High-energy rays are used to kill cancer cells or keep them from growing.
- **Chemotherapy**: Use of drugs to kill cancer cells or stop them from dividing.
- **Targeted Therapy**: Drugs or other substances that specifically target cancer cells without harming normal cells.
- **Immunotherapy**: Stimulates the body's immune system to fight the cancer.

Financial Implications:

Direct Medical Costs

- **Initial Diagnosis**: Costs associated with diagnostic tests can be substantial. Biopsies, imaging tests, and consultations with specialists may range from $1,000 to $5,000 or more.
- **Surgery**: The cost of surgical treatment can vary widely based on the complexity of the procedure and the hospital where it is performed. Surgery for oral cancer can range from $10,000 to $50,000 or more.
- **Radiation Therapy**: The total cost of radiation therapy can range from $10,000 to $50,000, depending on the number of treatments required.
- **Chemotherapy**: The cost of chemotherapy can vary greatly but typically ranges from $1,000 to $30,000 per month, depending on the drugs used and the length of treatment.
- **Follow-Up Care**: Continuous follow-up care is essential to monitor for recurrence and manage side effects, which adds to the long-term cost.

Indirect Costs

- **Lost Income**: Patients may need to take extended time off work for treatment and recovery, leading to loss of income.
- **Travel and Accommodation**: Costs for traveling to and from treatment centers, as well as potential accommodation if treatment is not available locally.
- **Supportive Care**: Costs for supportive treatments such as physical therapy, nutritional support, and psychological counseling.

Impact on Quality of Life:

- **Functional Impairments**: Treatment for oral cancer can result in significant functional impairments, such as difficulty in speaking, eating, and swallowing, which may require additional medical interventions and supportive care.
- **Aesthetic Changes**: Surgical treatments may lead to changes in appearance, necessitating reconstructive surgery or prosthetics, adding to the overall cost.

Prevention and Early Detection:

- **Avoid Tobacco and Limit Alcohol**: The most effective way to reduce the risk of oral cancer is to avoid all forms of tobacco and limit alcohol consumption.
- **HPV Vaccination**: Vaccination against HPV can significantly reduce the risk of HPV-related oral cancers.
- **Regular Dental Check-Ups**: Regular visits to the dentist for comprehensive exams and cleanings can help in early detection of precancerous conditions or early-stage cancer.

- **Self-Examinations**: Regular self-examinations for any unusual changes in the mouth can aid in early detection.

To carry out a mouth self-examination test the following will be required:

1. Mirror
2. Clean Fingers
3. Good Light source

During each stage, carefully examine and palpate for any irregularities such as lumps, red or white patches, alterations in color or texture, persistent ulcers, or any other abnormalities.

Face
Examine your entire face. Do you notice any new swellings? Check your skin for any recent changes. Have any moles increased in size or started to itch or bleed? Turn your head from side to side to stretch the skin over the muscles, making it easier to spot any lumps.

Neck
Using the pads of your fingers, run them beneath your jaw and along the large muscles on either side of your neck. Make sure you are not detecting any swellings. Or something with a different texture or consistent.

Lips
Utilize your index, middle fingers, and thumb to explore the interior of your mouth. Gently lift your upper lip upward and lower lip downward to examine for any sores or alterations in color. Employ your thumb and forefinger to carefully palpate both inside and around your lips, searching for any irregularities such as lumps, bumps, or changes in texture.

Gums
Using your thumb and forefinger, palpate both the inner and outer surfaces of the gums, systematically moving around to detect any abnormalities.

Check your Cheeks

Open your mouth and gently pull your cheeks away, one side at a time, using your finger to inspect the interior. Search for any red or white patches. Inside the cheek, use your finger to examine for ulcers, lumps, or tenderness. Repeat the process on the opposite side. Additionally, your tongue can assist in identifying sore spots, ulcers, or rough patches.

Tongue

Gently extend your tongue outward and examine one side before the other. Observe for any swelling, ulcers, or changes in color. To inspect the underside of your tongue, raise the tip of your tongue toward the roof of your mouth.

Floor of Mouth

Raise your tongue and inspect its underside, then examine the floor of your mouth for any abnormal color changes. Using gentle pressure, run your finger along the floor of your mouth and under your tongue to palpate for any lumps, swellings, or ulcers.

Roof of Mouth (Palate)

Tilt your head back and open your mouth widely to inspect the roof of your mouth. Look for any alterations in color or the presence of ulcers. Use your finger to assess changes in texture.

Take note of any unusual findings. If you've recently experienced a cold, sore throat, ulcer, swollen glands, or accidentally bitten or burned yourself, these issues typically resolve within three weeks. However, if you have any concerns, it's advisable to consult your dentist or doctor for potential specialized guidance.

6

Dental Treatments: Understanding Your Options and Making Informed Decisions

Navigating Dental Treatments: Understanding Your Options and Making Informed Decisions

Most common treatments and their financial costs

Knowing the most common oral treatments and their associated costs can help individuals plan and manage their dental care effectively. This chapter explores various common oral treatments, their purposes, and their financial implications.

Routine Preventive Care

Dental Cleanings and Check-up

Routine dental cleanings and check-ups are essential for maintaining oral health. These visits typically involve professional cleaning to remove plaque and tartar, oral cancer screenings, and thorough examinations to detect early signs of dental issues.

Professional cleanings, or prophylaxis, are essential for removing plaque and tartar build-up that regular brushing and flossing cannot eliminate. During a cleaning, a dental hygienist will:

Dental Cleaning

Remove Plaque and Tartar: Using specialized tools, hygienists clean above and below the gum line to remove hardened deposits that can cause gum disease.

Polish Teeth: Polishing smooths the tooth surface, making it more difficult for plaque to accumulate.

Check-ups

Regular dental check-ups, typically recommended every six months, are essential for early detection and prevention of oral health issues. During these visits, a dentist will:

Examine Teeth and Gums: Dentists look for signs of tooth decay, gum disease, and other oral health issues. Early detection allows for prompt treatment, preventing more severe problems.

Oral Cancer Screening: A vital part of the check-up, screening for oral cancer involves examining the mouth for any signs of cancerous or precancerous conditions.

Evaluate Bite and Jaw: Dentists check the alignment of teeth and jaws, looking for signs of issues like TMJ disorders.

Cost: The average cost for a dental cleaning and exam ranges from $75 to $200 without insurance. With insurance, most or all of the cost is often covered, especially if the visit is within the network and falls under preventive care.

Restorative Treatments

Fillings

Fillings are one of the most common dental procedures, essential for repairing teeth damaged by decay, wear, or minor fractures. Here we will see the various types of restorative fillings, the procedures involved, their benefits, and associated costs, providing a comprehensive overview for individuals considering this treatment.

What Are Restorative Fillings?

Restaurative fillings are materials used to fill cavities or repair damage to teeth. They restore the tooth's shape, function, and appearance, preventing further decay and maintaining overall oral health. The choice of filling material depends on the location of the cavity, the extent of the decay, patient preference, and cost considerations.

Types of Restorative Fillings

Amalgam Fillings

Amalgam fillings, also known as silver fillings, are made from a mixture of metals, including silver, mercury, tin, and copper. They have been used for over a century due to their durability and strength, this type of fillings have stood the test of time as a reliable, durable, and cost-effective dental restoration option. While concerns about mercury content persist, the consensus among health organizations is that they are safe for most individuals.

They have been a staple in restorative dentistry for over 150 years. Despite the advent of newer materials, amalgam fillings are still widely used today due to their proven track record and specific benefits.

Advances in dental materials have provided better options, allowing patients and dentists to choose the best solution based on individual needs, preferences, and economic considerations. Amalgam fillings continue to play a vital role in dental care worldwide, particularly for patients requiring a low cost treatment.

Pros:

- Long-lasting and durable
- Less expensive compared to other materials
- Strong and able to withstand chewing forces

Cons:

- Noticeable due to their metallic color
- Potential concerns about mercury content, although deemed safe by major health organizations

Cost: Amalgam fillings range from $50 to $150 per tooth.

Composite Resin Fillings

Composite resin fillings, or tooth-colored fillings, are made from a mixture of plastic and fine glass particles. They can be closely matched to the natural color of teeth, making them a popular choice for visible areas. It have become increasingly popular in modern dentistry due to their aesthetic appeal and versatility.

They are restorative materials used to repair cavities, minor fractures, and other damage to teeth. They are applied in layers and hardened using a special curing light, allowing for a precise and durable restoration that blends seamlessly with the natural tooth

While composite resin fillings are not as long-lasting as amalgam fillings, they can still provide many years of service with proper care. Typically, composite fillings last between 5 to 10 years. Advances in composite materials continue to improve their durability and resistance to wear.

Composite fillings are widely used in contemporary dental practice for both restorative and cosmetic purposes. They are the most used treatment for tooth decay and structural problems.

Unlike amalgam, composite resins fillings have an adhesive capability that enhances their performance and durability. One of their main advantages compared to amalgam restorations is that they do not require extensive removal of healthy tooth structure.

Pros:

- Aesthetically pleasing, as they blend with natural teeth
- Bond well to tooth structure, providing additional support
- Versatile and can be used for various types of restorations

Cons:

- May not be as durable as amalgam fillings, especially for large cavities
- More expensive than amalgam fillings
- Can take longer to place due to the bonding process

Cost: Composite resin fillings range from $90 to $250 per tooth.

Ceramic

Also known as porcelain fillings or ceramic inlays/onlays, are a popular choice in restorative dentistry due to their aesthetic appeal and durability. Made from high-quality dental ceramics, these fillings are designed to blend seamlessly with natural teeth while providing robust, long-lasting restorations.

Ceramic are used to repair teeth damaged by cavities, fractures, or wear. Unlike metal fillings, ceramic are made from porcelain, which mimics the natural appearance of tooth enamel. They can be used for **inlays**, which fit within the grooves of the tooth, **onlays**, which cover a larger portion of the tooth's surface, or **full crowns**, that replaces the entire crown structure of the tooth.

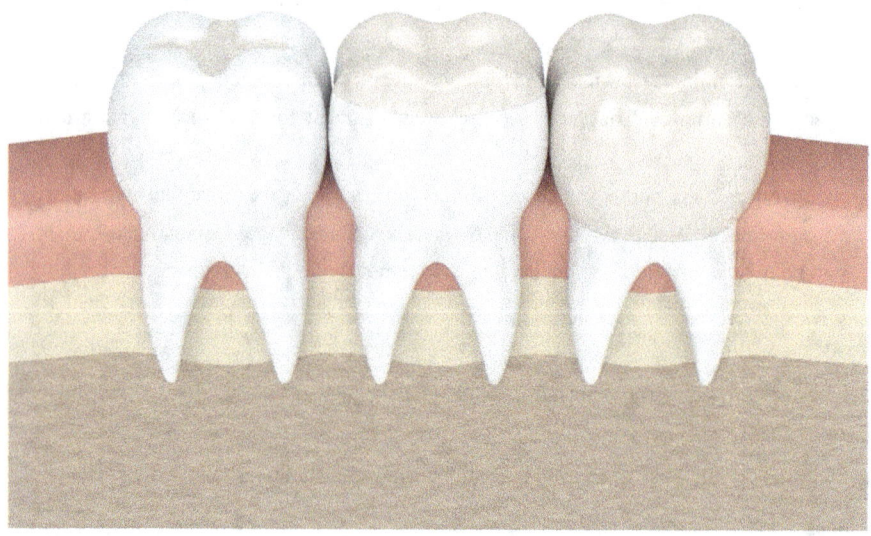

It represent a premium option in dental restorations, combining aesthetic excellence with durability and biocompatibility. Despite their higher cost and the potential need for multiple visits, they offer significant advantages, particularly for visible areas of the mouth where appearance is crucial. Patients considering ceramic fillings should discuss their options with their dentist to determine the best solution for their dental needs, ensuring a healthy and beautiful smile for years to come.

Pros:

- Highly aesthetic and natural-looking
- Resistant to staining
- Durable and long-lasting

Cons:

- More expensive than composite and amalgam fillings
- Requires more than one visit to place if fabricated in a lab

Cost: Ceramic fillings range from $250 to $4,500 per tooth, depending on the complexity and whether a lab is involved in creating the filling.

Glass Ionomer Fillings

Glass ionomer fillings are a unique type of dental restorative material known for their beneficial properties and specific applications. These fillings are made from a blend of glass and acrylic, providing certain advantages that make them particularly suitable for **pediatric dentistry** and specific clinical situations. This article delves into the characteristics, benefits, applications, and considerations of glass ionomer fillings in modern dental practice.

Glass ionomer fillings are restorative materials used to fill cavities and repair minor tooth damage. They were first introduced in the 1970s and have since become a valuable tool in dentistry. These fillings are composed of a silicate glass powder and a water-soluble polymer, creating a material that can bond chemically to the tooth structure without the need for a bonding agent.

Pros:

- Release fluoride, which helps protect the tooth from further decay
- Bond well to tooth structure
- Aesthetic appearance, although not as natural-looking as composite fillings

Cons:

- Less durable and more prone to wear and fractures
- Not suitable for areas subject to heavy chewing forces

Cost: Glass ionomer fillings range from $100 to $250 per tooth.

The Filling Procedure

1. **Diagnosis and Preparation**:

- The dentist diagnoses the cavity using visual inspection, X-rays, or other diagnostic tools.
- Local anesthesia is administered to numb the area around the affected tooth.

1. **Decay Removal**:

- The decayed portion of the tooth is removed using a drill or laser.
- The area is cleaned to ensure all decay and debris are eliminated.

1. **Filling Placement**:

- The filling material is placed in layers, with each layer being hardened using a special light (for composite fillings).
- For amalgam fillings, the material is placed directly into the cavity and shaped.
- For Ceramic, the material is bonded directly to the prepared teeth.

1. **Shaping and Polishing**:

- Once the filling is placed, the dentist shapes it to fit the tooth's contours.
- The filling is then polished to ensure a smooth surface that aligns with the bite.

Root Canals

Root canal treatment, also known as endodontic therapy, is a common dental procedure used to save teeth that are severely infected or damaged. This treatment involves removing the infected pulp from the tooth, cleaning and disinfecting the root canals, and then filling and sealing the space. This article provides an in-depth look at root canal treatment, including its purpose, procedure, benefits, and post-treatment care.

A root canal is a treatment designed to eliminate infection from the inner part of the tooth, known as the pulp. The pulp contains nerves, blood vessels, and connective tissue, and can become infected due to deep decay, repeated dental procedures, cracks, or trauma to the tooth.

The primary purpose of a root canal is to save a tooth that would otherwise need to be extracted. By removing the infected or damaged pulp, the procedure prevents the infection from spreading to other parts of the mouth and maintains the natural tooth's structure and function.

The Root Canal Procedure

Root canal treatment typically involves the following steps:

Diagnosis and Preparation: The dentist or endodontist takes X-rays to assess the extent of the infection and the shape of the root canals. Local anesthesia is administered to numb the area around the affected tooth.

Access Opening
A small opening is made in the crown of the tooth to access the pulp chamber and root canals.

Pulp Removal
The infected or damaged pulp is removed using specialized instruments called files. The root canals are thoroughly cleaned and disinfected to remove any remaining bacteria.

Shaping and Filling
The cleaned root canals are shaped and then filled with a biocompatible material called gutta-percha. This material seals the canals and prevents future infections

Sealing the Tooth
The access opening is sealed with a temporary or permanent filling. In many cases, a crown is placed over the tooth to restore its shape, strength, and function.

Follow-Up
A follow-up visit may be necessary to ensure the tooth is healing properly and to place a permanent restoration if a temporary filling was used initially.

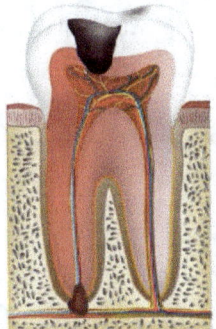

1. Infected tooth with abscess in the root

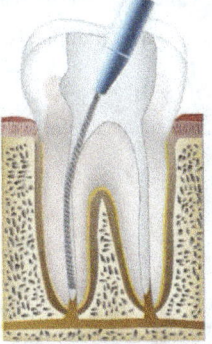

2. Files are used to clean out the infection

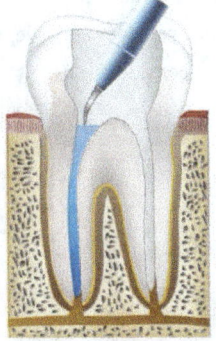

3. Canals are washed and dried

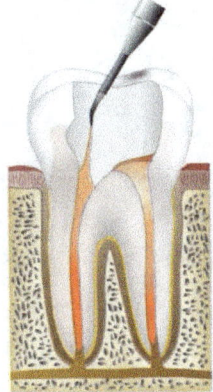

4. Canals filled with gutta percha

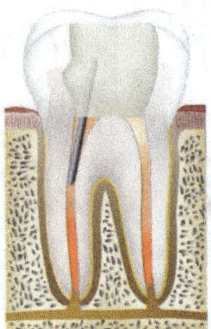

5. Opening sealed with filling, in some cases a post inserted to support crown

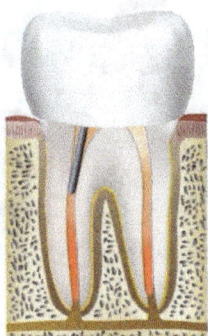

5. Crown cemented onto rebuild tooth

One of the advantages of root canal treatment is the relief of pain, which is usually incredibly severe. Although the main purpose is to avoid removing the tooth so that the patient does not have to replace it with dental replacement options, which are much more expensive and have a significant impact on their financial health.

Cost: Root canals can be costly, ranging from $700 to $1,500 for front teeth and $1,000 to $2,000 for molars. The price varies based on the tooth's location and the complexity of the procedure.

Tooth Replacement Options

Dental Implants

Dental implants are a revolutionary solution for replacing missing teeth, offering a durable, functional, and aesthetically pleasing alternative to traditional dentures and bridges. This article provides an in-depth look at dental implants, including their benefits, procedure, types, and considerations.

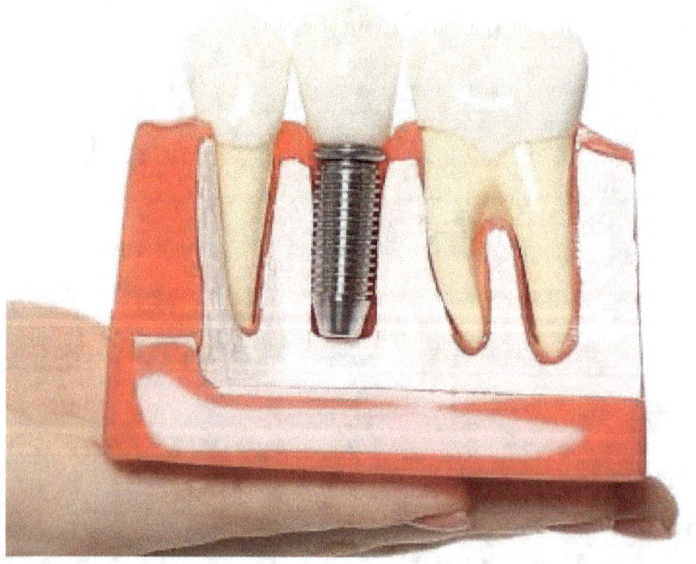

Dental implants are artificial tooth roots made of biocompatible materials, typically titanium, that are surgically placed into the jawbone. These implants serve as a stable foundation for fixed or removable replacement teeth, which are designed to match the natural teeth.

1	Initial Consultation	2	Treatment Planning	3	Bone Grafting (if necessary)
	The process begins with a thorough examination and consultation with a dentist or oral surgeon. This includes dental X-rays and impressions to assess bone structure and plan the treatment.		Based on the assessment, a customized treatment plan is created. This plan considers the number of implants needed, the condition of the jawbone, and the desired outcome.		If there is insufficient bone to support the implant, a bone graft may be required. This procedure involves adding bone material to the jawbone to ensure a stable foundation for the implant.
4	Implant Placement	5	Abutment Placement	6	Crown Placement
	During the surgical procedure, the dental implant is placed into the jawbone. This is typically done under local anesthesia, though sedation may be used for patient comfort. The implant is then left to integrate with the bone, a process called osseointegration, which takes several months.		Once the implant has integrated with the bone, a small connector called an **abutment** is attached to the implant. This abutment will hold the replacement tooth or crown.		After the gums have healed, a custom-made crown is attached to the abutment. This crown is designed to blend seamlessly with the natural teeth in terms of shape, size, and color.

Implants are a highly effective and versatile solution for replacing missing teeth, whether you need to replace a single tooth or multiple teeth. They provide a durable, natural-looking, and functional replacement, enhancing both oral health and overall quality of life.

Replacing a Single Tooth

When a single tooth is missing, a dental implant is an excellent option for replacement.
Procedure:
- **Implant Placement**: A titanium implant is surgically placed into the jawbone where the missing tooth's root was located.
- **Osseointegration**: Over a few months, the implant fuses with the jawbone through a process called osseointegration, creating a solid foundation.

- **Abutment and Crown**: After osseointegration, an abutment (connector) is attached to the implant, and a custom-made crown is placed on top. This crown is designed to match the shape, size, and color of your natural teeth.

Benefits:
- **Preserves Adjacent Teeth**: Unlike traditional bridges, a single implant does not require the alteration of adjacent teeth.
- **Prevents Bone Loss**: The implant stimulates the jawbone, preventing the bone loss that typically occurs with missing teeth.
- **Restores Function and Appearance**: The implant looks and functions like a natural tooth, allowing for normal eating and speaking.

Replacing Multiple Teeth

When we want to replace more than one tooth, we can use the multiple implants technique. In this technique, we use two or more implants to support more than two teeth, using the implants as pillars, like a bridge. With two implants, we can rehabilitate up to 6 teeth. In more complex cases, we use 4 implants to rehabilitate an entire arch.

Implant-Supported Bridges:
- **Procedure**: Instead of placing an implant for every missing tooth, a few strategically placed implants can support a bridge. For example, if three teeth are missing in a row, two implants can support a bridge that replaces all three teeth.
- **Benefits**: This reduces the number of implants needed while still providing stability and preserving jawbone health.

All-on-4 or All-on-6 Implants:

In some cases, we need to use dental implants to rehabilitate more than one tooth. In these cases, we can us a technique called all-on-4, where we restore an entire arch with just 4 implants. This type of treatment can restore the patient's chewing, aesthetics, speech, and self-esteem in as little as 3 days.

- **Procedure**: This technique uses four or six implants to support a full arch of teeth, either upper, lower, or both.
- **Benefits**: This method is cost-effective and less invasive than placing individual implants for each missing tooth. It provides a full set of permanent, stable teeth that function like natural teeth.

Cost: Dental implants are expensive, with costs ranging from $1,500 to $6,000 per implant. This cost includes the implant, abutment, and crown but can increase if additional procedures like bone grafting are required.

Dentures

Dentures are removable dental appliances designed to replace missing teeth and restore function, aesthetics, and overall oral health. They come in various types and styles to suit different needs and preferences. This article explores the different types of dentures, their benefits, the fitting process, and important care considerations.

Types of Dentures

1. **Complete Dentures**: Also known as full dentures, these are used when all teeth in the upper or lower jaw are missing. They consist of a full set of artificial teeth attached to an acrylic base that resembles the gum tissue.
2. **Partial Dentures**: These are used when some natural teeth remain. Partial dentures consist of replacement teeth attached to a gum-colored base, often connected by a metal framework that holds the denture in place in the mouth

Cost: The cost of dentures varies widely. Complete dentures can range from $1,000 to $3,000 per arch, while partial dentures range from $500 to $1,500. The price can increase based on the materials used and additional treatments required for fitting.

Cosmetic Treatments

Teeth Whitening

Teeth whitening has become a popular cosmetic dental procedure, offering individuals a safe and effective way to enhance the appearance of their smile. This article explores the process of teeth whitening, its benefits, different methods available, and important considerations for achieving a brighter, more confident smile.

Teeth whitening may not be effective on dental restorations such as crowns, veneers, or fillings. These materials do not respond to bleaching agents in the same way as natural teeth and may require replacement to match the new tooth shade.

However, it offers a simple yet effective way to achieve a brighter, more confident smile. Whether through professional in-office treatments or at-home whitening kits prescribed by a dentist, individuals can enjoy the benefits of a whiter smile and improved self-esteem. With proper care and maintenance, teeth whitening can provide long-lasting results, allowing individuals to smile with confidence and radiate positivity in all aspects of life.

This cosmetic dental procedure effectively removes stains and discoloration, resulting in a whiter and more radiant smile. Let's delve into the details of teeth whitening, including the methods, benefits, and considerations.

How Teeth Whitening Works

Teeth whitening works by bleaching the enamel of the teeth to lighten their color. There are two primary methods of teeth whitening:

In-Office Professional Whitening:

- **Procedure**: This method involves a visit to the dentist, where a professional-strength bleaching agent is applied to the teeth. The dentist may use a special light or laser to enhance the whitening effect.
- **Benefits**: In-office whitening produces immediate and dramatic results, often lightening teeth by several shades in a single session. The procedure is supervised by a dental professional, ensuring safety and effectiveness.

At-Home Whitening Kits:

- **Procedure**: At-home whitening kits typically consist of custom-fitted trays and a bleaching gel. The trays are filled with the gel and worn over the teeth for a specified period, usually several hours each day or overnight.
- **Benefits**: At-home whitening kits offer convenience and flexibility, allowing users to whiten their teeth at their own pace and in the comfort of their home. While results may take longer to achieve compared to in-office treatment, they can still be significant with consistent use.

Benefits of Teeth Whitening

- **Enhanced Appearance**: Teeth whitening can dramatically improve the brightness and attractiveness of your smile, boosting your confidence and self-esteem.
- **Youthful Appearance**: Whiter teeth are often associated with youthfulness and vitality, making you appear younger and more vibrant.

- **Minimal Invasive Procedure**: Compared to other cosmetic dental procedures, teeth whitening is relatively non-invasive and does not require altering the structure of the teeth.
- **Quick Results**: In-office whitening can produce immediate results, while at-home kits can deliver noticeable improvements within a few weeks of regular use.

Considerations and Precautions

While teeth whitening is generally safe and effective, there are some considerations and precautions to keep in mind:

- **Potential Sensitivity**: Some individuals may experience temporary tooth sensitivity or gum irritation during or after whitening treatment. Using desensitizing toothpaste or reducing the frequency of whitening sessions can help alleviate discomfort.
- **Not Suitable for Everyone**: Teeth whitening may not be suitable for individuals with certain dental conditions, such as cavities, gum disease, or intrinsic discoloration. A dental consultation is recommended to determine candidacy for whitening treatment.
- **Maintenance Required**: To maintain results, regular touch-up treatments may be necessary, especially for individuals who consume staining beverages or foods or use tobacco products.

Teeth whitening is a popular and effective way to achieve a brighter, more youthful smile. Whether you opt for in-office professional whitening or at-home whitening kits, the result is a noticeable improvement in the appearance of your teeth and a boost in confidence. However, it's essential to consider the potential risks and consult with a dental professional before undergoing whitening treatment to ensure safety and optimal results. With proper care and maintenance, you can enjoy a dazzling smile that radiates health and vitality for years to come.

Cost: Professional teeth whitening costs range from $300 to $800 per session. Over-the-counter options are cheaper but generally less effective, costing between $20 and $100.

Veneers

Veneers are thin, custom-made shells crafted from durable materials like porcelain or composite resin. These shells are bonded to the front surface of teeth to improve their appearance, correcting issues such as discoloration, chips, cracks, or misalignment. Let's delves into the details of veneers, including their benefits, the procedure involved, types available, and important considerations for those considering this cosmetic dental treatment.

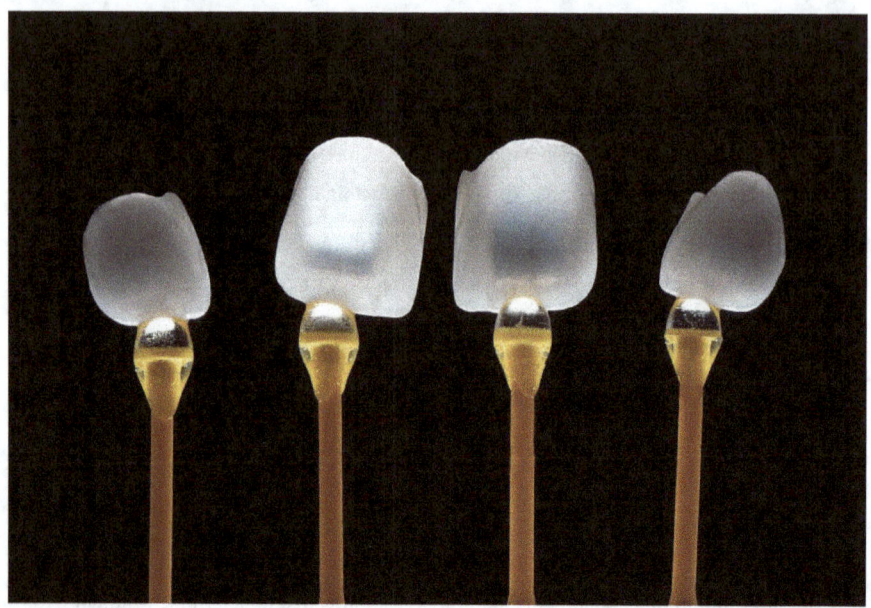

Veneers provide a long-term solution for individuals looking to enhance the appearance of their teeth. Custom-made to fit each individual's unique smile, veneers offer a natural and seamless result. However, it is important to consider factors such as cost, maintenance, and potential for future replacement when deciding if veneers are the right option for you.

Understanding Veneers

Veneers are a versatile cosmetic dental solution designed to enhance the aesthetics of a smile. They can address various imperfections in teeth, including:

Stains and Discoloration
Veneers can cover stains that are resistant to teeth whitening treatments, restoring a bright, white appearance

Chips and Cracks
Veneers can repair minor chips and cracks in teeth, improving their overall shape and symmetry

Gaps and Spaces
Veneers can close gaps between teeth, creating a more uniform and balanced smile

Misalignment
Veneers can visually straighten the appearance of slightly crooked or misaligned teeth, providing a more harmonious smile

Benefits of Veneers

Natural Appearance: Veneers are custom-made to match the color, shape, and size of natural teeth, resulting in a seamless and lifelike appearance.

Versatility: Veneers can address multiple cosmetic concerns with a single treatment, offering a comprehensive solution for smile enhancement.

Minimal Tooth Preparation: Unlike crowns, which require significant tooth reduction, veneers involve minimal removal of tooth structure, preserving more of the natural tooth.

Stain Resistance: Porcelain veneers are highly resistant to stains from food, beverages, and tobacco, maintaining their brightness and translucency over time.

Durable and Long-lasting: With proper care, veneers can last for many years, providing lasting improvements to the smile.

The Veneer Placement Process

1. **Initial Consultation**: The process begins with a consultation with a cosmetic dentist to discuss goals, expectations, and suitability for veneers. X-rays and impressions may be taken to assess the teeth and plan the treatment.
2. **Preparation**: A small amount of enamel is removed from the front surface of the teeth to make room for the veneers. This step is minimal but essential for ensuring a natural-looking result and proper bonding of the veneers.
3. **Impressions**: Impressions of the prepared teeth are taken to create custom veneers that fit precisely over the teeth and complement the patient's smile.
4. **Temporary Veneers**: Temporary veneers may be placed to protect the prepared teeth while the permanent veneers are being fabricated in a dental laboratory. These temporary veneers provide a preview of the final result.
5. **Bonding**: Once the permanent veneers are ready, they are bonded to the teeth using a strong dental adhesive. The dentist carefully positions each veneer and adjusts the fit as needed for optimal comfort and aesthetics.
6. **Final Touches**: Any final adjustments are made to ensure the veneers blend seamlessly with the natural teeth and provide a comfortable bite.

Types of Veneers

- **Porcelain Veneers**: Made from high-quality dental porcelain, porcelain veneers offer exceptional durability, aesthetics, and stain resistance. They are custom-made in a dental laboratory for precise fit and natural appearance.
- **Composite Veneers**: Composite veneers are made from tooth-colored composite resin material applied directly to the teeth and shaped by the dentist. While more affordable than porcelain veneers, composite veneers may not last as long and are more prone to staining and wear.

Cost: The cost of veneers ranges from $800 to $2,500 per tooth. Porcelain veneers are typically more expensive than composite resin veneers.

7

Oral Health for Different Life Stages

Oral health is important at every stage of life, from infancy to old age. Here are some key tips for maintaining good oral health at each life stage:

Infancy and Early Childhood: Building a Foundation for Lifelong Oral Health

Oral health is crucial in infancy and early childhood as it sets the foundation for lifelong dental health. Proper oral hygiene practices should begin as soon as the first tooth erupts, usually around six months of age. It is important for parents and caregivers to clean their child's gums and teeth regularly to prevent tooth decay and other dental issues.

During infancy, parents can use a soft, damp cloth or gauze to gently clean the baby's gums after feedings. Once teeth start to erupt, a small, soft-bristled toothbrush should be used with a tiny smear of fluoride toothpaste. Be as the child grows, the amount of toothpaste can be increased to a pea-sized amount.

Be careful, we should only use fluoride toothpaste after your baby learns how to spit. If your child ingests too much fluoride, they may develop a condition called fluorosis, which is a change in dental enamel caused by excessive fluoride intake.

Regular dental check-ups are also important during infancy and early childhood to monitor the growth and development of the child's teeth and to catch any potential issues early on. The American Academy of Pediatrics recommends that children see a dentist by their first birthday or within six months of the first tooth erupting.

In addition to proper oral hygiene practices, it is important for parents to be mindful of their child's diet and nutrition. Limiting sugary snacks and drinks can help prevent tooth decay and cavities. Encouraging healthy eating habits and providing a balanced diet can also contribute to good oral health.

Teething can be a challenging time for both infants and parents, as it may be accompanied by discomfort, irritability, and excessive drooling. Parents can alleviate teething discomfort by gently massaging the infant's gums with a clean finger or providing teething rings or toys to chew on.

Over-the-counter teething gels or medications containing benzocaine should be used with caution due to potential safety concerns, and caregivers should consult with a healthcare provider before using them.

Preventing Early Childhood Caries (ECC)

Early childhood caries, also known as baby bottle tooth decay, is a significant concern during infancy and early childhood. It occurs when sugary liquids, such as milk or juice, pool around the teeth for extended periods, leading to tooth decay.

To prevent ECC, caregivers should avoid putting infants to bed with bottles containing sugary liquids and limit their consumption of sugary snacks and drinks. If you find it difficult to prevent your baby from falling asleep after a bottle of milk or breastfeeding before bedtime, you can use a moist cloth to gently clean your baby's mouth after feeding

Overall, establishing good oral health habits early on in infancy and early childhood can set the stage for a lifetime of healthy smiles. By practicing good oral hygiene, visiting the dentist regularly, and promoting a healthy diet, parents can help ensure their child's teeth and gums stay strong and healthy for years to come.

Tips for Infancy and childhood:
1. Clean your baby's gums with a damp cloth after feedings.
2. Once teeth start to come in, brush them with a soft baby toothbrush and a small amount of fluoride toothpaste.
3. Limit sugary snacks and drinks, as they can contribute to tooth decay.
4. Schedule your child's first dental visit before their first birthday.

Adolescence, taking care of your oral health can be fun!

Adolescence is a crucial time for oral health, as this is when permanent teeth have fully emerged and there may be a greater risk of cavities, gum disease, and other oral health issues. It is important for adolescents to establish good oral hygiene habits to maintain a healthy smile for a lifetime.

During adolescence, hormonal changes can increase the risk of gum disease, so it is important for teenagers to brush and floss regularly to prevent plaque buildup and keep their gums healthy. Regular dental check-ups and cleanings are also essential to catch any issues early and prevent them from progressing.

Adolescents may also be at risk for dental injuries, especially if they participate in sports or other physical activities. Wearing a mouthguard can help protect their teeth from trauma and prevent costly dental treatments down the road.

It is also important for adolescents to be mindful of their diet and avoid sugary snacks and drinks that can contribute to tooth decay. Encouraging them to drink plenty of water and eat a balanced diet rich in fruits and vegetables can help support good oral health.

Overall, taking care of oral health during adolescence is crucial for maintaining a healthy smile and preventing long-term dental issues. By establishing good oral hygiene habits early on, adolescents can enjoy a lifetime of healthy teeth and gums.

Also, it is worth mentioning that regular visits to the dentist remain highly important during this time of life, as it is typically a period when the patient may require corrective treatments such as orthodontic and orthopedic appliances. During this stage of life, orthodontic treatments can be more effective than in an adult patient.

Tips for Adolescence

1. Emphasis on establishing good oral hygiene routines, including brushing three times a day and flossing regularly.
2. Wear a mouthguard during sports to protect your teeth from injury
3. Importance of fluoride in preventing tooth decay and strengthening enamel.
4. Discussion of common oral health issues during adolescence, such as orthodontic problems and wisdom teeth eruption.

Adulthood, prevention is the key.

Maintaining good oral health is important at every stage of life, but it becomes even more crucial as we age. As we reach adulthood, our risk for oral health issues such as tooth decay, gum disease, and tooth loss increases. This is due to a combination of factors, including changes in our bodies as we age, the effects of medications, medical conditions, and lifestyle habits.

One common issue that adults may face is gum disease, also known as periodontal disease. This condition occurs when bacteria in the mouth cause inflammation and infection in the gums, leading to symptoms such as redness, swelling, bleeding, and bad breath. If left untreated, gum disease can progress to more severe forms and even result in tooth loss.

Tooth decay is another common issue that adults may experience. This can be caused by a variety of factors, including poor oral hygiene, a diet high in sugary and acidic foods, and a lack of regular dental check-ups. Cavities can lead to pain, infection, and the need for costly dental treatments such as fillings or root canals.

In addition to gum disease and tooth decay, adults may also be at risk for other oral health issues such as dry mouth, oral cancer, and tooth sensitivity. It is important to be proactive about maintaining good oral hygiene habits, including brushing and flossing regularly, eating a healthy diet, avoiding tobacco products, and visiting the dentist for regular check-ups and cleanings.

By taking care of our oral health as adults, we can help prevent these issues and maintain a healthy smile for years to come. Remember, a healthy mouth is a key component of overall health and well-being.

Tips for Adulthood

1. Continue to brush and floss regularly, and see your dentist for regular check-ups and cleanings.
2. Wear a mouthguard during sports to protect your teeth from injury.
3. Limit sugary and acidic foods and drinks, as they can contribute to tooth decay and erosion.
4. Avoid smoking and using tobacco products, as they can harm your oral health.
5. Consider dental treatments such as teeth whitening or straightening if desired.

Older adulthood, how to enjoy your well cared oral health.

As we age, maintaining good oral health becomes increasingly important. Older adults are more susceptible to dental problems such as gum disease, tooth decay, and oral infections. These issues can be exacerbated by factors such as dry mouth, medication side effects, and chronic health conditions.

As the population continues to age, the importance of oral health for seniors becomes increasingly important. Seniors are a special patient population with unique oral health needs that must be addressed in order to maintain overall health and quality of life.

One of the most common oral health issues that seniors face is dry mouth, also known as xerostomia. This condition can be caused by a variety of factors, including medications, certain medical conditions, and the natural aging process. Dry mouth can lead to a host of oral health problems, such as tooth decay, gum disease, and oral infections. It is important for seniors to stay hydrated and to speak with their healthcare provider about any medications that may be causing dry mouth.

Another common oral health issue for seniors is tooth decay. As we age, our teeth become more susceptible to decay due to factors such as receding gums, weakened enamel, and decreased saliva production. Seniors should continue to brush and floss regularly, as well as visit their dentist for regular check-ups and cleanings. In some cases, seniors may benefit from the use of fluoride treatments or prescription-strength toothpaste to help prevent tooth decay.

Gum disease is another common oral health issue that affects seniors. Gum disease is caused by the buildup of plaque and tartar on the teeth, which can lead to inflammation and infection of the gums. If left untreated, gum disease can progress to more serious conditions such as periodontitis, which can result in tooth loss. Seniors should practice good oral hygiene habits, such as brushing and flossing regularly, and should visit their dentist for regular cleanings and check-ups to prevent gum disease.

Seniors are also more likely to experience tooth loss as they age. Tooth loss can have a significant impact on a person's quality of life, affecting their ability to eat, speak, and smile with confidence. In addition to maintaining good oral hygiene habits, seniors can also benefit from the use of dentures or dental implants to replace missing teeth and restore their smile. It is important for seniors to discuss their tooth replacement options with their dentist to determine the best treatment plan for their individual needs.

In addition to these common oral health issues, seniors may also be at increased risk for oral cancer. Oral cancer can be caused by a variety of factors, including smoking, excessive alcohol consumption, and sun exposure. Seniors should be aware of the signs and symptoms of oral cancer, such as persistent mouth sores, difficulty chewing or swallowing, and changes in the appearance of the lips or mouth. Routine oral cancer screenings during dental check-ups can help detect abnormalities early and improve treatment outcomes. Educating seniors about the signs and symptoms of oral cancer, such as mouth sores, persistent mouth pain, and difficulty swallowing, is essential for early detection and intervention.

Many seniors take multiple medications to manage chronic health conditions, some of which can have adverse effects on oral health. Certain medications may cause dry mouth, gum overgrowth, or increased susceptibility to dental decay. Dentists and healthcare providers should be aware of seniors' medication regimens and monitor for any oral health-related side effects.

Mobility limitations and other physical disabilities can make it challenging for seniors to maintain proper oral hygiene practices. Caregivers and family members can assist seniors with oral care tasks, such as brushing and flossing, or consider adaptive devices such as electric toothbrushes or floss picks to facilitate oral hygiene routines.

Promoting good oral health in seniors requires a multi-faceted approach that addresses the unique needs of this population. In addition to practicing good oral hygiene habits, seniors can also benefit from a healthy diet rich in fruits and vegetables, which can help to maintain overall health and prevent oral health issues. Seniors should also avoid tobacco use and limit their alcohol consumption, as these habits can increase the risk of oral health problems.

Regular visits to the dentist are essential for seniors to maintain good oral health. Dentists can provide preventive care, such as cleanings and check-ups, as well as treat any oral health issues that may arise. Seniors should also discuss any concerns or changes in their oral health with their dentist, as early detection and treatment can help to prevent more serious problems from developing.

Older adults should also be mindful of their diet and nutrition, as what we eat can have a significant impact on our oral health. Eating a balanced diet rich in fruits, vegetables, and lean proteins can help to keep teeth and gums healthy. Avoiding sugary and acidic foods and beverages can also help to prevent tooth decay and gum disease.

For older adults who wear dentures or implants, it is important to clean and care for them properly to prevent infections and discomfort. Dentures should be removed and cleaned daily, and individuals should also make sure to clean their gums and any remaining natural teeth. As for implants, they need to be cleaned properly and require regular maintenance with your dentist.

Overall, maintaining good oral health at an older age is crucial for overall health and well-being. By practicing good oral hygiene, visiting the dentist regularly, and eating a healthy diet, older adults can help to prevent dental problems and maintain a healthy smile for years to come.

In conclusion, seniors are a special patient population with unique oral health needs that must be addressed in order to maintain overall health and quality of life. By practicing good oral hygiene habits, staying hydrated, and visiting the dentist regularly, seniors can promote and maintain good oral health well into their golden years. It is important for seniors to be proactive about their oral health and to seek treatment for any oral health issues that may arise. By taking care of their oral health, seniors can enjoy healthy smiles and improved quality of life as they age.

Tips for Seniors:
1. Continue to brush and floss regularly, and be vigilant for signs of gum disease or other oral health issues.
2. Consider using a fluoride toothpaste or mouthwash to help prevent tooth decay.
3. Be aware of any changes in your oral health, such as dry mouth or tooth sensitivity, and discuss them with your dentist.

Pregnancy

Pregnancy is a time of significant physical and hormonal changes that can affect a woman's oral health. Understanding the unique oral health considerations during pregnancy is essential for maintaining good oral hygiene and overall well-being for both the mother and the baby.

Pregnancy is a special time in a woman's life, filled with excitement and anticipation. However, it is also a time when a woman's body undergoes significant changes, including hormonal fluctuations that can affect her oral health. Pregnant women are at an increased risk of developing oral health problems, such as gum disease and tooth decay, due to these hormonal changes.

Maintaining good oral health is important for pregnant women, not only for their own well-being but also for the health of their developing baby. Poor oral health has been linked to an increased risk of preterm birth and low birth weight, as well as other complications during pregnancy.

One of the most common oral health problems experienced by pregnant women is gum disease, also known as gingivitis. This condition is characterized by red, swollen, and bleeding gums, and is caused by the buildup of plaque on the teeth. Hormonal changes during pregnancy can make gums more sensitive to plaque, leading to an increased risk of gingivitis.

Gum bleeding during pregnancy is a common concern that many expectant mothers experience. It is often due to hormonal changes that occur during pregnancy, particularly an increase in progesterone levels. These hormonal fluctuations can lead to an exaggerated response of the gums to plaque bacteria, resulting in inflammation and bleeding, a condition known as pregnancy gingivitis

In addition to gum disease, pregnant women are also at risk of developing tooth decay. This is due to a combination of factors, including increased cravings for sugary foods and drinks, as well as morning sickness that can lead to vomiting and acid erosion of the teeth. Furthermore, hormonal changes can also affect the bacteria in the mouth, increasing the risk of cavities.

Morning sickness, characterized by frequent vomiting during early pregnancy, can have detrimental effects on oral health. The stomach acids brought up during vomiting can erode tooth enamel, leading to increased tooth sensitivity, decay, and gum irritation. It's essential for pregnant individuals experiencing morning sickness to take steps to minimize the impact on their oral health, such as rinsing the mouth with water after vomiting and using fluoride toothpaste to help strengthen tooth enamel.

It is important for pregnant women to take extra care of their oral health during this time. This includes brushing and flossing regularly, using a fluoride toothpaste, and visiting the dentist for regular check-ups and cleanings. In some cases, a pregnant woman may need to see a periodontist, a dentist who specializes in treating gum disease, for more advanced treatment.

Pregnant women should also be aware of the importance of a healthy diet for their oral health. Eating a balanced diet that is low in sugar and high in nutrients can help to prevent gum disease and tooth decay. It is also important to drink plenty of water to help wash away food particles and bacteria from the mouth.

In addition to maintaining good oral health habits, pregnant women should also be aware of the potential risks of certain dental treatments during pregnancy. While routine dental cleanings and check-ups are generally safe, some treatments, such as X-rays and certain medications, should be avoided during pregnancy. It is important for pregnant women to inform their dentist of their pregnancy and discuss any concerns or questions they may have about dental treatment.

Oral health is an important aspect of prenatal care for pregnant women. By taking care of their oral health during pregnancy, women can reduce the risk of developing gum disease and tooth decay, and improve their overall well-being. Pregnant women should work closely with their dentist to ensure that they are receiving the best possible care for their oral health during this special time in their lives.

In summary:

- **Hormonal Changes:** During pregnancy, hormonal fluctuations, particularly increased levels of estrogen and progesterone, can affect the oral cavity. These hormonal changes can lead to an increased risk of gingivitis (gum inflammation), gum sensitivity, and even pregnancy tumors (non-cancerous growths on the gums).
- **Morning Sickness and Acid Erosion:** Many pregnant women experience morning sickness, which can result in frequent vomiting and acid reflux. The acidic stomach contents can erode tooth enamel, leading to increased tooth sensitivity and a higher risk of cavities. Rinsing the mouth with water or a fluoride mouthwash after vomiting can help neutralize acids and protect the teeth.
- **Pregnancy Gingivitis:** Gingivitis, or inflammation of the gums, is a common oral health concern during pregnancy. Hormonal changes make the gums more susceptible to irritation from plaque bacteria, leading to red, swollen, and tender gums. Practicing good oral hygiene, including brushing and flossing regularly, can help prevent and manage pregnancy gingivitis.
- **Increased Risk of Periodontal Disease:** Untreated gingivitis can progress to periodontal disease, a more severe form of gum disease that can lead to tooth loss

and other health complications. Pregnant women with periodontal disease may be at higher risk of adverse pregnancy outcomes, such as preterm birth and low birth weight. Seeking professional dental care and treating gum disease during pregnancy is crucial for both maternal and fetal health.

- **Dental Visits During Pregnancy:** Routine dental care, including dental cleanings and check-ups, is safe and recommended during pregnancy. However, it's essential to inform your dentist of your pregnancy and any changes in your health status. Some elective dental procedures may be postponed until after delivery, while essential treatments can be performed safely with appropriate precautions

Overall, maintaining good oral health at every life stage involves regular brushing and flossing, limiting sugary and acidic foods and drinks, and seeing your dentist for regular check-ups and cleanings. By prioritizing your oral health throughout your life, you can help prevent tooth decay, gum disease, and other oral health issues

8

Oral Health Myths and Facts

Oral health is an important aspect of overall well-being, yet there are many myths and misconceptions surrounding this topic. In this chapter, we will debunk some common myths and provide evidence-based facts to help you maintain optimal oral health.

Myth #1: Brushing harder will clean your teeth better.

Fact: Brushing too hard can actually damage your teeth and gums. Dentists recommend using a soft-bristled toothbrush and gentle brushing motions to effectively clean your teeth without causing harm. Brushing too hard can wear down enamel, injure your gums and lead to tooth sensitivity, increasing the risk of cavities.

Myth #2: You only need to see a dentist if you have a toothache.

Fact: Regular dental check-ups are essential for maintaining good oral health. Dentists can detect early signs of dental issues such as cavities, gum disease, and oral cancer. By visiting your dentist regularly, you can prevent small problems from becoming larger and more costly to treat.

Myth #3: Sugar is the main cause of cavities.

Fact: While sugar can contribute to the development of cavities, it is not the only factor, the bacteria that cause cavities don't just feed on sugar. They also feed on any other food debris lodged in the teeth, gums, or tongue, or even on dead cells that have been shed from the tissue in your mouth.. Poor oral hygiene, bacteria in the mouth, and acidic foods and drinks can also play a role in cavity formation. It is important to brush and floss regularly, limit sugary foods and drinks, and maintain a balanced diet to prevent cavities.

Myth #4: You only need to floss when food gets stuck between your teeth.

Fact: Flossing should be a daily part of your oral hygiene routine. Flossing helps remove plaque and food particles from between your teeth and along the gumline, where your toothbrush cannot reach. By flossing regularly, you can prevent cavities, gum disease, and bad breath.

Myth #5: Mouthwash can replace brushing and flossing.

Fact: Mouthwash is not a substitute for brushing and flossing. While mouthwash can help freshen your breath and kill bacteria in your mouth, it does not remove plaque or food particles. Brushing three times a day and flossing once a day are essential for maintaining good oral hygiene.

Myth #6: Baby teeth are not important because they will eventually fall out.

Fact: Baby teeth play a crucial role in a child's oral health. Baby teeth help children chew food, speak clearly, and hold space for permanent teeth to come in properly. Neglecting baby teeth can lead to dental issues such as cavities, infections, and misalignment of permanent teeth.

Myth #7: You should avoid going to the dentist during pregnancy.

Fact: It is safe to visit the dentist during pregnancy, and in fact, it is important to maintain good oral health during this time. Pregnancy hormones can increase the risk of gum disease and tooth decay, so regular dental check-ups are essential for preventing oral health issues.

Myth #8: You should brush your teeth immediately after eating.

Fact: Brushing immediately after eating acidic foods or drinks can actually damage your teeth. Acid softens the enamel, and brushing right away can wear it down further. Dentists recommend waiting at least 30 minutes after eating before brushing to allow your saliva to neutralize acids in your mouth.

Myth #9: You do not need to see a dentist if you have dentures.

Fact: Even if you have dentures, it is important to see a dentist regularly for check-ups and adjustments. Dentures can cause irritation, sores, and changes in the mouth's shape over time. A dentist can ensure that your dentures fit properly and address any oral health issues that may arise.

Myth #10: You cannot prevent gum disease.

Fact: Gum disease is preventable with good oral hygiene habits. Brushing three times a day, flossing once a day, and visiting your dentist regularly can help prevent gum disease. Early signs of gum disease, such as red or swollen gums, bleeding when brushing, and bad breath, should not be ignored.

Myth#11: Brushing teeth immediately before a dental appointment will hide poor oral hygiene habits.

Fact: Dentists can often tell if someone has neglected their oral hygiene regardless of whether they brush right before an appointment. Regular oral care is essential for maintaining oral health.

Myth#12: Dental treatments are always painful.

Fact: Modern dental techniques and anesthesia make most dental procedures relatively painless. Dentists prioritize patient comfort and use various methods to minimize discomfort during treatments.

Myth#13: Dental x-rays are harmful and should be avoided.

Fact: Dental x-rays emit low levels of radiation and are considered safe when necessary for diagnosing dental problems. Dentists use lead aprons and modern equipment to minimize radiation exposure.

Myth#14: Wisdom teeth cause crowding of other teeth.

Fact: Wisdom teeth may contribute to crowding in some cases, but often there are other factors involved, such as genetics and improper oral hygiene.

Myth#15: You can't get cavities if you have dental sealants.

Fact: While dental sealants provide an extra layer of protection against cavities, they don't guarantee immunity. Proper oral hygiene and regular dental visits are still necessary.

Myth#16: Natural toothpaste is always better than conventional toothpaste.

Fact: While some natural toothpaste options are effective, not all of them contain fluoride, which is crucial for preventing cavities. Always check the label for fluoride content.

Myth#17: Chewing sugar-free gum is as effective as brushing.

Fact: While sugar-free gum can stimulate saliva production and help clean teeth between meals, it doesn't replace the thorough cleaning provided by brushing and flossing.

Myth#18: Fluoride in toothpaste is harmful.

Fact: Fluoride in toothpaste helps prevent cavities and strengthen tooth enamel. When used as directed, fluoride toothpaste is safe and beneficial for oral health. We should only be cautious when using fluoride in babies who have not yet learned to spit, as ingesting high concentrations of fluoride can cause a health issue called fluorosis.

Myth#19: You should avoid brushing bleeding gums.

Fact: Brushing gently can actually help improve gum health by removing plaque. Bleeding gums may indicate gingivitis, and regular brushing and flossing can help alleviate it.

Myth#20: Dental implants are guaranteed to last a lifetime.

Fact: While dental implants are durable and long-lasting, their longevity depends on factors such as oral hygiene, lifestyle habits, and overall health. Proper care and regular dental check-ups are essential for maintaining implant health.

There are many myths and misconceptions surrounding oral health. By understanding the facts and following evidence-based practices, you can maintain optimal oral health and prevent dental issues. Remember to brush and floss regularly, visit your dentist for check-ups, and follow a balanced diet to keep your teeth and gums healthy.

9

Oral Health on a budget

Preventive measures to maintain a healthy mouth

Implementing a comprehensive preventive care strategy is crucial for maintaining a healthy mouth and saving money on dental expenses. This includes regular brushing and flossing, using fluoride products, and scheduling routine dental check-ups and cleanings. By addressing issues early and keeping your mouth in optimal condition, you can avoid the need for more extensive and costly treatments down the line.

Brush Three times a Day
Brush your teeth for two minutes, twice a day, using a soft-bristled toothbrush and fluoride toothpaste. This helps remove plaque and prevent the development of cavities and gum disease.

Floss Daily
Flossing once a day helps remove food particles and plaque from areas your toothbrush can't reach, reducing the risk of gum disease and tooth decay.

Use Fluoride Products
Incorporating fluoride into your oral hygiene routine, such as using fluoride toothpaste, can strengthen tooth enamel and prevent the formation of cavities.

Schedule Regular Dental Visits
Visit your dentist for a professional cleaning and comprehensive exam every 6 months. This allows them to catch any issues early and provide preventive care to keep your mouth healthy.

How preventive measures can you save money?

Preventive measures are key to saving money on oral health care. By taking proactive steps to maintain good oral hygiene, you can avoid costly dental procedures down the road. One of the most effective preventive measures is regular brushing and flossing. By brushing your teeth at least three times a day and flossing daily, you can remove plaque and bacteria that can lead to tooth decay and gum disease. This simple routine can save you hundreds, if not thousands, of dollars in dental bills.

Another important preventive measure is regular dental check-ups. By seeing your dentist for routine cleanings and exams, you can catch any potential problems early on before they escalate into more serious issues. This can help you avoid costly treatments such as fillings, root canals, and extractions. Additionally, some dental insurance plans cover preventive care at little to no cost, making it a cost-effective way to maintain good oral health.

In addition to regular brushing, flossing, and dental check-ups, a healthy diet can also play a role in saving money on oral health care. Consuming foods high in sugar and carbohydrates can increase your risk of tooth decay and gum disease, leading to expensive dental treatments. By incorporating more fruits, vegetables, and whole grains into your diet, you can improve your oral health and reduce your risk of dental problems.

Furthermore, avoiding harmful habits such as smoking and excessive alcohol consumption can also save you money on oral health care. These habits can increase your risk of oral cancer, gum disease, and tooth loss, all of which can result in costly treatments. By quitting smoking and moderating your alcohol intake, you can improve your oral health and potentially save money on dental bills in the long run.

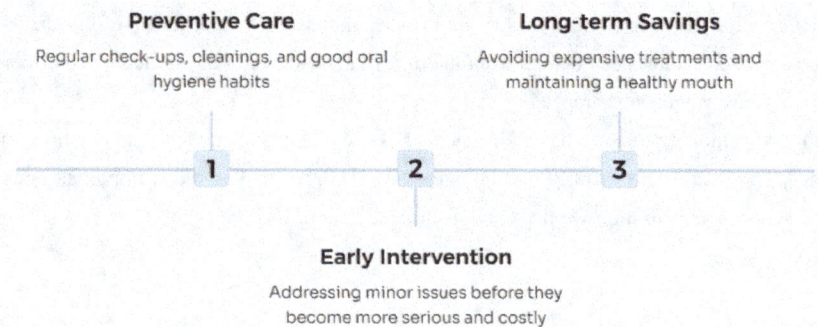

Here is a list of habit you should avoid:

Smoking

Smoking weakens the immune system in the mouth, making it harder for the body to fight off bacteria and infections. This weakens the gums and makes them more susceptible to gum disease. Smokers are more likely to develop periodontal disease, characterized by inflammation, gum recession, bone loss, and eventually tooth loss.

It also impairs blood flow to the gums and oral tissues, which slows down the healing process after dental procedures or oral surgery. This can lead to complications such as dry socket after tooth extraction and delayed healing of oral wounds.

The tar and nicotine in tobacco smoke stain teeth, giving them a yellowish or brownish appearance. Smokers are also more likely to suffer from chronic bad breath (halitosis) due to the presence of tobacco particles and chemicals in the mouth.

Smoking decreases saliva production in the mouth, leading to dry mouth (xerostomia). Saliva helps wash away food particles, neutralize acids, and remineralize tooth enamel. Without adequate saliva, smokers are at a higher risk of tooth decay and oral infections.

Perhaps the most serious consequence of smoking is the increased risk of oral cancer. Tobacco smoke contains numerous carcinogens (cancer-causing agents) that can damage DNA and lead to the development of cancerous lesions in the mouth, including on the lips, tongue, cheeks, and throat. Smokers are at a much higher risk of developing oral cancer compared to non-smokers, and the risk increases with the duration and intensity of smoking.

It can compromise the success of various dental treatments, such as dental implants, root canal therapy, and periodontal treatment. Reduced blood flow and impaired healing in smokers may lead to higher failure rates and complications following dental procedures.

Smoking accelerates the aging process in the mouth, leading to premature wrinkling around the lips (smoker's lines), loss of gum tissue, and a sunken appearance of the cheeks. These cosmetic changes can detract from the overall appearance of the smile and contribute to a prematurely aged appearance.

Overall, smoking tobacco poses significant risks to oral health and can lead to a range of serious oral health problems. Quitting smoking is one of the most important steps individuals can take to improve their oral health and overall well-being.

Excessive sugar

Sugars from foods and beverages feed the bacteria that naturally reside in the mouth. These bacteria metabolize sugars and produce acids as byproducts. Over time, these acids can erode tooth enamel, leading to the formation of dental plaque, a sticky film of bacteria and food particles that adheres to the teeth.

The acids produced by bacteria in dental plaque attack tooth enamel, causing demineralization and eventually leading to tooth decay (cavities). The longer sugars remain in contact with the teeth, the greater the risk of decay. Foods and beverages high in sugars, such as candy, soda, and sweets, are particularly harmful to dental health when consumed frequently or in large quantities.

In addition to promoting bacterial growth, sugary foods and beverages themselves can be acidic, further contributing to enamel erosion. Acidic foods and drinks weaken tooth enamel and make it more susceptible to decay. Citrus fruits, fruit juices, and sports drinks are examples of acidic beverages that can erode tooth enamel when consumed excessively.

Sugary foods and beverages can also contribute to gum disease (gingivitis and periodontitis) by fueling bacterial growth along the gumline. Bacteria in dental plaque produce toxins that irritate the gums, leading to inflammation, swelling, and bleeding. If left untreated, gum disease can progress to more severe forms and result in gum recession, bone loss, and tooth loss.

Poor oral health resulting from excessive sugar consumption has been linked to various systemic health issues, including diabetes, cardiovascular disease, and respiratory infections. Bacteria from the mouth can enter the bloodstream and contribute to inflammation and other health problems throughout the body.

Excessive sugar consumption during childhood is particularly concerning, as it can lead to the early development of dental caries and set the stage for poor oral health throughout life. Parents and caregivers should be mindful of the sugar content in children's diets and encourage healthy eating habits from a young age to promote optimal oral health.

To mitigate the negative effects of sugar on oral health, individuals should limit their consumption of sugary foods and beverages, practice good oral hygiene habits (such as brushing twice a day, flossing daily, and visiting the dentist regularly), and choose nutritious foods that promote dental health. Additionally, drinking water after consuming sugary foods or beverages can help rinse away sugars and acids from the mouth, reducing their harmful effects on teeth.

Nail biting and Biting Hard Objects

Biting down on hard objects, such as ice, pens, or fingernails, can exert excessive force on the teeth, leading to fractures or chips. Teeth are designed for chewing food, not for biting into hard objects. When subjected to significant force, teeth can sustain structural damage that may require dental treatment to repair.

Habitual biting on hard objects or nails can cause abrasion and wear on tooth enamel over time. Enamel is the outermost layer of the tooth that protects against decay and sensitivity. When enamel wears down, teeth become more susceptible to damage, decay, and sensitivity.

Excessive biting on hard objects or nails can expose the underlying dentin, a softer layer of the tooth beneath the enamel. Dentin contains tiny tubules that connect to the nerves of the tooth. When dentin is exposed, it can lead to increased tooth sensitivity to hot, cold, sweet, or acidic foods and beverages.

Habitual nail biting or biting on hard objects can place stress on the temporomandibular joint (TMJ), the joint that connects the jawbone to the skull. Over time, this repetitive stress can contribute to TMJ disorders, characterized by symptoms such as jaw pain, clicking or popping sounds in the jaw, difficulty opening or closing the mouth, and headaches.

Biting nails introduces harmful bacteria from the hands and nails into the mouth, increasing the risk of oral infections and gum disease. Bacteria can easily enter small cuts or abrasions around the nails and transfer to the oral cavity, where they can proliferate and cause inflammation and infection.

Chronic nail biting or biting on hard objects can lead to unsightly changes in the appearance of the teeth and surrounding tissues. For example, persistent nail biting can cause irregularities in the shape or length of the nails, while biting on hard objects can result in chipped, worn, or fractured teeth that detract from the overall aesthetic of the smile.

To address these harmful habits and protect oral health, individuals should make a conscious effort to avoid biting on hard objects or nails. Employing stress-reduction techniques, such as deep breathing, exercise, or mindfulness practices, can help reduce the urge to engage in these habits. Additionally, individuals may benefit from using bitter-tasting nail polish or wearing a mouthguard to discourage nail biting or teeth grinding. Seeking support from a dentist or mental health professional may also be beneficial for breaking these habits and promoting optimal oral health.

Mouthguard

Sports-related dental injuries, such as broken or knocked-out teeth, fractured jaws, and soft tissue injuries, are common among athletes who do not wear mouthguards. Impact from collisions, falls, or contact with equipment or other players can cause serious damage to the teeth and surrounding structures in the mouth.

Mouthguards act as a protective barrier between the teeth, lips, cheeks, tongue, and soft tissues of the mouth and the hard surfaces encountered during sports activities. They absorb and distribute the force of impact, reducing the risk of dental trauma and minimizing the severity of injuries.

It helps cushion and stabilize the teeth, preventing them from hitting against each other or against the jaws during impact. This reduces the likelihood of tooth fractures, chips, or avulsions (complete displacement from the socket) that may occur in the event of a collision or fall.

In addition to safeguarding the teeth, mouthguards may also help reduce the risk of concussions and traumatic brain injuries by absorbing and dispersing the forces of impact that can jolt the head and neck during sports-related collisions or falls.

Athletes who have undergone dental procedures such as braces, bridges, implants, or cosmetic dentistry rely on mouthguards to protect their investment in dental work. Without proper protection, these dental appliances and restorations are vulnerable to damage during sports activities.

Mouthguards not only shield the teeth but also provide a cushioning effect for the lips, cheeks, tongue, and gums, reducing the risk of lacerations, bruises, and other soft tissue injuries that may result from accidental blows or impacts to the face.

Incorporating mouthguard use into sports safety practices helps raise awareness about the importance of oral health protection among athletes, coaches, and parents. By prioritizing mouthguard use, individuals can take proactive measures to safeguard their smiles and prevent unnecessary dental injuries.

Overall, wearing a properly fitted mouthguard is essential for protecting oral health and minimizing the risk of sports-related dental injuries. Athletes of all ages and skill levels should prioritize mouthguard use during sports activities to ensure their smiles remain healthy and intact.

Teeth Griding (Bruxism)

Persistent teeth grinding can lead to excessive wear and tear on the tooth enamel. Over time, this can result in flattened, chipped, fractured, or sensitive teeth. The constant pressure and friction exerted on the teeth during grinding can weaken their structure and increase the risk of dental problems such as cavities and cracks.

Bruxism can strain the muscles, ligaments, and joints that control jaw movement, leading to temporomandibular joint (TMJ) disorders. Symptoms of TMJ disorders may include jaw pain, stiffness, clicking or popping sounds in the jaw, difficulty opening or closing the mouth, and headaches. Chronic teeth grinding can exacerbate TMJ symptoms and contribute to ongoing discomfort and dysfunction in the jaw joint.

Individuals who grind their teeth may experience facial pain, tension, or soreness, particularly in the jaw, temples, or surrounding muscles. The repetitive muscle contractions associated with bruxism can lead to muscle fatigue, inflammation, and discomfort in the face and neck area.

Grinding can wear down the protective enamel layer of the teeth, exposing the underlying dentin and increasing tooth sensitivity to hot, cold, sweet, or acidic foods and beverages. In severe cases, bruxism may contribute to tooth fractures, particularly in teeth that have been weakened by previous dental work or decay.

The excessive forces exerted on the teeth and surrounding tissues during grinding can contribute to gum recession, where the gum tissue pulls away from the teeth, exposing the tooth roots. Gum recession can increase tooth sensitivity and raise the risk of gum disease (periodontitis), as the roots become more susceptible to bacterial plaque and tartar buildup.

It often occurs during sleep, and individuals may be unaware of their grinding habits until they experience symptoms such as jaw pain or tooth sensitivity. Chronic teeth grinding can disrupt sleep patterns and lead to fatigue, daytime drowsiness, and other sleep-related issues.

It is often associated with stress, anxiety, tension, or other emotional factors. Individuals may unconsciously clench or grind their teeth as a coping mechanism for stress or as a manifestation of underlying psychological distress. Addressing stress through relaxation techniques, counseling, or stress management strategies may help alleviate bruxism symptoms.

Overall, teeth grinding can have detrimental effects on oral health and overall well-being. Seeking professional dental care is essential for diagnosing and managing bruxism effectively, and treatment options may include wearing a custom-fitted mouthguard (night guard), stress management techniques, muscle relaxation exercises, behavior modification strategies, and addressing underlying factors contributing to bruxism. Early intervention can help prevent further damage to the teeth and jaws and promote optimal oral health outcomes.

Brushing the teeth too harshly

Aggressive brushing can damage the delicate gum tissue, leading to gum recession. When gums recede, the roots of the teeth become exposed, increasing the risk of tooth sensitivity, decay, and gum disease. Receding gums also give the teeth a longer appearance and can affect the overall aesthetics of the smile.

Brushing too hard can wear down the protective enamel layer of the teeth, exposing the underlying dentin. Dentin contains microscopic tubules that connect to the nerve endings of the tooth, making it more sensitive to hot, cold, sweet, or acidic stimuli. Individuals who brush aggressively may experience increased tooth sensitivity and discomfort.

Abrasion typically occurs at the gumline or on the surfaces of the teeth near the gumline, where the enamel is thinner. Over time, tooth abrasion can result in irreversible damage and increase the risk of cavities, cracks, and fractures.

Aggressive brushing can injure the soft tissues of the mouth, including the gums, cheeks, lips, and tongue. Forceful brushing motions may cause irritation, inflammation, and even minor cuts or abrasions in the oral mucosa. These injuries can be painful and may increase the risk of oral infections.

Brushing with excessive force can accelerate the wear and tear of toothbrush bristles. Over time, the bristles may become frayed, flattened, or splayed, reducing their effectiveness in removing plaque and debris from the teeth. Inadequate plaque removal can lead to plaque buildup, tartar formation, and oral health problems.

Aggressive brushing can compromise the integrity of dental restorations, such as fillings, crowns, bridges, and veneers. Excessive force applied to these restorations may cause them to loosen, chip, crack, or become dislodged prematurely. Individuals with dental work should exercise caution when brushing to avoid damaging their restorations.

Your brushing habits can perpetuate a cycle of oral health problems and reinforce harmful behaviors. Individuals who brush forcefully may inadvertently cause damage to their teeth and gums, leading to discomfort or sensitivity that prompts them to brush even harder in an attempt to clean their teeth more thoroughly.

To promote optimal oral health, individuals should brush their teeth gently yet thoroughly using a soft-bristled toothbrush and a fluoride toothpaste. Using gentle, circular motions and holding the toothbrush at a 45-degree angle to the gumline can help remove plaque effectively without causing damage to the teeth or gums. Additionally, scheduling regular dental check-ups and cleanings can help identify and address any oral health issues before they progress.

Ultimately, by addressing oral health issues early and maintaining good hygiene habits, you can avoid the need for more extensive and expensive treatments down the line. Regular check-ups and cleanings allow your dentist to identify and address problems before they become more serious, potentially saving you thousands of dollars in the long run. Additionally, proper brushing, flossing, and the use of fluoride can help prevent the development of cavities and other oral health issues, reducing your overall dental expenses.

10

Mastering the Basics: Essential Oral Hygiene Practices

Proper brushing and flossing techniques are essential for maintaining good oral health down the road. By practicing these simple habits on a daily basis, you can keep your teeth and gums healthy . In this subchapter, we will discuss the importance of proper brushing and flossing techniques

Maintaining good oral hygiene habits can go a long way in preventing costly dental problems. Simple practices like brushing three times a day, flossing daily, and using fluoride toothpaste can help keep your mouth healthy. Regular dental check-ups and cleanings are also crucial, as they allow your dentist to catch any issues early, coach you about **Oral Health Education** and provide preventive care.

Brushing

Brush your teeth three times a day for two minutes each time using a soft-bristled toothbrush and fluoride toothpaste. Proper brushing technique is key to removing plaque and preventing cavities.

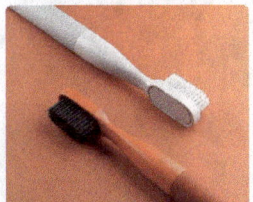

Flossing

Flossing once a day helps remove food particles and plaque from areas your toothbrush can't reach, reducing the risk of gum disease and tooth decay.

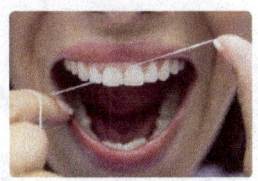

Regular Dental Visits

Schedule a professional cleaning and exam every 6 months. Your dentist can identify and treat any issues early, preventing them from becoming more serious and costly.

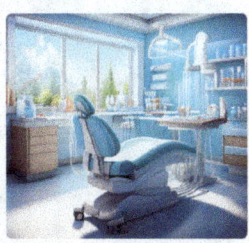

Brushing

When it comes to brushing your teeth, it's important to use a soft-bristled toothbrush and fluoride toothpaste. Brush your teeth at least three times a day, making sure to brush for a full two minutes each time. Be sure to brush all surfaces of your teeth, including the front, back, and chewing surfaces. It's also important to brush your tongue to remove bacteria and freshen your breath. By following these simple steps, you can effectively remove plaque and prevent cavities and gum disease.

Brushing your teeth effectively involves a few key steps:

- **Choose the Right Toothbrush:** Use a toothbrush with soft bristles that fits comfortably in your mouth and can reach all areas easily.
- **Use Fluoride Toothpaste:** Apply a **pea-sized amount** of fluoride toothpaste to your toothbrush. Fluoride helps strengthen tooth enamel and prevent tooth decay.
- **Brush at a 45-Degree Angle:** Hold your toothbrush at a 45-degree angle to your gums. This helps clean both the teeth and the gumline.
- **Brush Gently:** Use gentle, circular motions to brush the outer surfaces, inner surfaces, and chewing surfaces of your teeth. Avoid brushing too hard, as this can damage your gums and enamel.
- **Don't Forget the Tongue:** Gently brush your tongue to remove bacteria and freshen your breath.
- **Brush for Two Minutes:** Aim to brush your teeth for at least two minutes each time, ensuring you thoroughly clean all surfaces.
- **Rinse Thoroughly:** After brushing, rinse your mouth thoroughly with water to remove any remaining toothpaste and debris.
- **Replace Your Toothbrush Regularly:** Replace your toothbrush every three to four months, or sooner if the bristles become frayed.

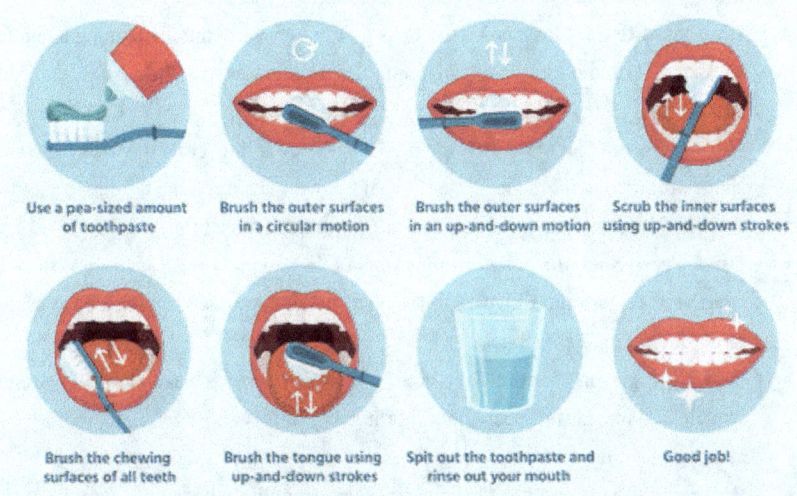

By following these steps and brushing your teeth at least twice a day, you can maintain good oral hygiene and prevent dental problems.

Flossing

In addition to brushing, flossing is also crucial for maintaining good oral health. Flossing helps remove food particles and plaque from between your teeth, where your toothbrush can't reach. To floss properly, use about 18 inches of floss and gently slide it between your teeth, making a C shape around each tooth. Be sure to floss all of your teeth, including the back ones. Flossing should be done at least once a day to prevent cavities and gum disease. I know flossing can sometimes feel tedious, but its cleaning contributes to about 2/5 of dental hygiene. So, if you skip flossing, it's like you're only doing half the job.

Here's how to floss your teeth effectively:

- **Choose Your Floss:** There are various types of dental floss available, including waxed, unwaxed, flavored, and floss picks. Choose one that you find comfortable to use.
- **Cut an Adequate Length:** Cut a piece of floss about 18 to 24 inches long. This allows you to use a fresh section of floss for each tooth.

- **Hold the Floss Properly:** Wrap the ends of the floss around your middle fingers, leaving about 1-2 inches of floss between them. Use your thumbs and index fingers to guide the floss between your teeth.
- **Gently Glide the Floss:** Slide the floss gently between your teeth using a gentle back-and-forth motion. Avoid snapping the floss into your gums, as this can cause irritation.
- **Curve Around Each Tooth:** As you reach the gum line, curve the floss into a C shape around one tooth and slide it up and down the side of the tooth. Be sure to go slightly beneath the gum line to remove plaque and debris.
- **Use a Fresh Section:** After cleaning one tooth, unwind a fresh section of floss from your fingers and move on to the next tooth. Continue this process for each tooth, including the back teeth.
- **Be Thorough but Gentle:** Take your time to floss between each tooth, ensuring you clean both sides of each tooth thoroughly. However, be gentle to avoid causing bleeding or irritation to your gums.
- **Rinse and Dispose:** After flossing, rinse your mouth with water to remove any loosened plaque and debris. Dispose of the used floss in the trash.

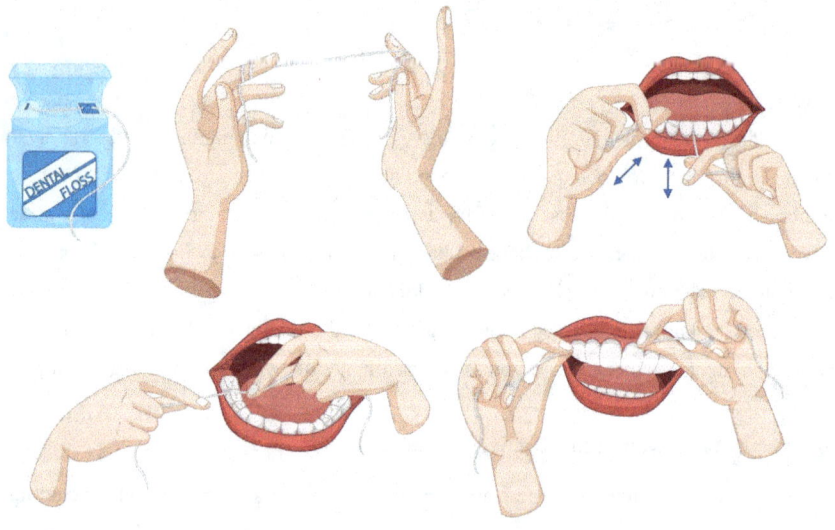

By flossing your teeth at least once a day, you can remove plaque and food particles from areas that your toothbrush can't reach, helping to prevent cavities, gum disease, and bad breath.

Regular Dental Visits

By visiting your dentist regularly, you can ensure that any dental issues are detected and treated early. Regular dental check-ups and cleanings are essential for maintaining good oral health and preventing future problems. Don't forget to schedule your next dental appointment!

Your dentist will be able to thoroughly clean your teeth, removing any plaque and tartar buildup that regular brushing and flossing may miss. Additionally, they will be able to perform a comprehensive examination of your mouth to check for any signs of dental problems. Don't neglect your dental health - make your next appointment today!

You can turn your dentist into an **Oral health coach** , that means your dentist can teach and monitor whether your oral cleaning technique is correct or insufficient. Also, your dentist can also teach you and give tips on how to identify problems in your oral health early on, so that you can identify the problem and schedule an appointment before it evolves.

By incorporating proper brushing and flossing techniques into your daily routine, you can save money on expensive dental procedures in the future. Regular dental cleanings and check-ups are important for maintaining good oral health, but by taking care of your teeth at home, you can reduce the frequency of these visits. Remember, prevention is key when it comes to oral health, and by practicing good oral hygiene habits, you can keep your mouth healthy and your wallet happy.

Be cautious with mouthwashes

Antiseptic mouthwashes can help reduce bacteria and prevent gum disease, but we should avoid alcohol-based mouthwashes, which can exacerbate dry mouth. Instead, we should look for alcohol-free

The oral health industry makes various products that, when used correctly, greatly aid in maintaining a good and healthy mouth. Unfortunately, in some cases, advertisements lead us to buy products that, if we used indiscriminately, can cause problems for our health. One example of these products is mouthwashes, which can cause health issues

Mouthwashes should be used to help control our bacterial flora when we have what we called a dysbiosis which is an imbalance in bacterial composition, changes in bacterial metabolic activities, or changes in bacterial distribution. In healthy patients, where we have a balance of these bacteria, mouthwash has no therapeutic action and ends up disrupting this balance, thus causing a problem of bacterial imbalance that can turn a healthy mouth into an unhealthy one.

Choosing the Right Oral Care Products Without Breaking the Bank

Taking care of your oral health doesn't have to break the bank. With so many oral care products on the market, it can be overwhelming to choose the right ones that are both effective and affordable.

When choosing oral care products, it is important to look for ones that have the American Dental Association (ADA) seal of approval. This seal indicates that the product has been tested and approved by dental professionals for safety and effectiveness. By selecting products with the ADA seal, you can ensure that you are using high-quality products that will help maintain good oral health without spending a lot of money.

Another tip for choosing affordable oral care products is to opt for store-brand options. Many store brands offer quality oral care products at a fraction of the cost of name-brand products. These products often contain the same active ingredients as their more expensive counterparts, making them a budget-friendly option for those looking to save money on oral care.Additionally, consider purchasing oral care products in bulk or during sales and promotions.

Lastly, buying in bulk can help you save money in the long run, while taking advantage of sales and promotions can help you score discounts on your favorite oral care products. By stocking up on essentials when they are on sale, you can save money without sacrificing the quality of your oral care routine.

Advanced Oral Care Techniques and Products

While regular brushing and flossing are essential components of a good oral hygiene routine, there are advanced techniques and products available that can enhance oral health even further. This section delves into innovative approaches to oral care and introduces advanced products designed to optimize dental hygiene.

Water Flossers

Water flossers, also known as oral irrigators, use a stream of water to clean between teeth and along the gumline. They are particularly beneficial for individuals with braces, implants, or bridges, as well as those who have difficulty using traditional floss. Water flossers can effectively remove plaque and debris, promoting healthier gums and reducing the risk of gum disease.

Water flossers, also known as oral irrigators or water picks, are advanced oral care devices that use a steady stream of water to remove plaque, food particles, and bacteria from between teeth and along the gumline. They offer an alternative or supplement to traditional flossing and can be particularly beneficial for individuals with orthodontic appliances, dental implants, or sensitive gums.

Here are some key features and benefits of water flossers:

Effective Plaque Removal: Water flossers utilize a pulsating or steady stream of water to dislodge plaque and debris from areas that are difficult to reach with traditional floss. The pressure of the water helps flush out bacteria and food particles, leaving the mouth feeling clean and refreshed.

Gentle on Gums: Water flossers provide a gentle yet thorough cleaning action that is less abrasive than traditional flossing. This makes them suitable for individuals with sensitive gums or those who find traditional flossing uncomfortable or difficult to perform.

Ideal for Orthodontic Appliances: People with braces, bridges, or dental implants often struggle to clean between teeth and around wires or brackets. Water flossers offer an effective solution for removing plaque and food debris from these hard-to-reach areas, helping to maintain oral health during orthodontic treatment.

Ideal for Implants hygiene: Patients with dental implants should use this tool to improve the hygiene of their implants. Dental implants require special care to avoid health issues and extend their longevity. To facilitate this hygiene or assist patients with motor problems, water flossers are an excellent option.

Customizable Settings: Many water flossers come with adjustable pressure settings, allowing users to customize the intensity of the water stream to their comfort level and oral health needs. This flexibility makes water flossers suitable for individuals of all ages and with varying degrees of oral sensitivity.

Improved Gum Health: Regular use of a water flosser can contribute to healthier gums by reducing inflammation, bleeding, and the risk of gum disease. The gentle massaging action of the water stimulates blood flow to the gums, promoting tissue health and overall gum health.**Convenient and Easy to Use:** Water flossers are user-friendly devices that are easy to operate and maintain. They typically feature reservoirs for water, adjustable pressure settings, and interchangeable tips for different cleaning needs. Many models also come with built-in timers to ensure users floss for the recommended amount of time.

Portability and Accessibility: Water flossers are available in a range of sizes and designs, including countertop models and cordless, portable units. This versatility makes them suitable for use at home, in the office, or while traveling, ensuring consistent oral care even when away from home.

Gum Massage

Gum massage is a simple yet effective technique that involves gently massaging the gums with your fingers to improve blood circulation and promote gum health. This technique can help reduce inflammation, prevent gum disease, and strengthen the gum tissue. To perform gum massage, use your index fingers to gently massage the gums in a circular motion for a few minutes. Gum massage can be done daily after brushing and flossing.

Interdental Brushes

Interdental brushes are small, disposable brushes designed to clean between teeth and around dental appliances. They come in various sizes to accommodate different interdental spaces and can be particularly useful for individuals with gaps, crowding, or orthodontic appliances. Interdental brushes complement traditional flossing by providing additional plaque removal in hard-to-reach areas.

Key Features and Benefits of Interdental Brushes

Interdental brushes are specifically designed to reach and clean the tight spaces between tooth where plaque and food particles often accumulate. Their small, bristled heads can effectively dislodge and remove debris, reducing the risk of cavities and gum disease.

They are user-friendly and can be easier to handle than traditional dental floss, especially for individuals with limited dexterity. They typically feature a short handle and a brush head that can be maneuvered into tight spaces with minimal effort.

Interdental brushes come in a range of sizes and shapes to accommodate different interdental spaces and dental conditions. This makes them versatile tools that can be used by individuals with gaps, crowding, or orthodontic appliances, as well as those with bridges, implants, or crowns.

Regular use of interdental brushes can help improve gum health by reducing inflammation and preventing gum disease. The gentle scrubbing action of the bristles massages the gums, promoting blood circulation and overall gum wellness.

Individuals with braces, retainers, or other orthodontic appliances often find it challenging to clean around wires and brackets with traditional floss. Interdental brushes can easily navigate these obstacles, ensuring thorough cleaning and reducing the risk of plaque buildup and gum disease during orthodontic treatment.

Interdental brushes are compact and portable, making them convenient for use at home, at work, or while traveling. Many brands offer travel-friendly cases or caps to keep the brushes clean and protected when not in use.

Using interdental brushes in conjunction with regular brushing and flossing provides a comprehensive approach to oral hygiene. They can help reach areas that a toothbrush or floss might miss, ensuring a more thorough clean and better overall oral health.

How to Use Interdental Brushes

1. **Choose the Right Size:** Select an interdental brush size that fits comfortably between your teeth without causing discomfort or damage to the gums. You may need different sizes for different areas of your mouth.
2. **Insert the Brush:** Gently insert the interdental brush between your teeth, close to the gumline. Do not force it; if the brush is too large, try a smaller size.
3. **Clean the Spaces:** Move the brush back and forth a few times in a horizontal motion to clean the space between your teeth. Make sure to cover all sides of the teeth and the gumline.
4. **Rinse the Brush:** Rinse the brush under running water to remove any debris and bacteria. If the brush head becomes worn or damaged, replace it with a new one.
5. **Repeat:** Use the interdental brush for all the spaces between your teeth, adjusting the size as needed for different areas.

Tips for Effective Use

- **Regular Use:** Incorporate interdental brushes into your daily oral hygiene routine, ideally after brushing your teeth.
- **Gentle Handling:** Be gentle when inserting and using the brush to avoid damaging your gums.
- **Professional Advice:** Consult your dentist or dental hygienist for recommendations on the appropriate size and technique for your specific dental needs.

Tongue Scrapers

Tongue scrapers are tools used to remove bacteria, food debris, and dead cells from the surface of the tongue. Cleaning the tongue can help improve breath freshness, reduce the risk of oral infections, and enhance overall oral hygiene. Tongue scrapers are available in plastic or metal designs and are easy to use as part of a daily oral care routine.Key Features and Benefits of Tongue Scrapers

One of the primary benefits of using a tongue scraper is its ability to combat bad breath (halitosis). The tongue's surface can harbor bacteria and food particles that contribute to foul odors. Regular scraping can reduce these bacteria, resulting in fresher breath.

A cleaner tongue can enhance your sense of taste. By removing the build-up of residue on the tongue, food flavors can be better perceived, making eating a more enjoyable experience.

The tongue is a breeding ground for bacteria, which can lead to various oral health issues, including tooth decay and gum disease. Using a tongue scraper helps to remove these bacteria, promoting better overall oral health.

Incorporating tongue scraping into your daily oral care routine can complement other practices like brushing and flossing. This comprehensive approach ensures that more areas of the mouth are kept clean, reducing the risk of dental problems.

Tongue scrapers are simple and quick to use. They come in various designs, including plastic or metal, and are designed to be gentle yet effective in removing debris from the tongue.

How to Use a Tongue Scraper

1. **Choose a Scraper:** Select a tongue scraper made from metal or plastic, depending on your preference. Ensure it has a comfortable handle and a smooth edge.
2. **Extend Your Tongue:** Stick out your tongue as far as possible to expose its surface.
3. **Scrape Gently:** Place the scraper at the back of your tongue and gently pull it forward toward the tip. Be careful not to scrape too hard to avoid irritating the tongue.
4. **Rinse the Scraper:** Rinse the scraper under running water to remove the debris and bacteria collected.
5. **Repeat as Necessary:** Repeat the scraping process 2-3 times or until your tongue feels clean. Rinse your mouth with water afterward.
6. **Clean the Scraper:** After use, thoroughly clean the scraper and store it in a hygienic place.

Tips for Effective Use

- **Use Daily:** Make tongue scraping a part of your daily oral hygiene routine, ideally in the morning to remove the overnight buildup.
- **Be Gentle:** Avoid pressing too hard to prevent irritation or injury to the tongue.
- **Stay Consistent:** Consistent use is key to experiencing the full benefits of tongue scraping.
- **Consult a Dentist:** If you have any concerns or experience discomfort, consult your dentist for advice.

Although adding tongue scraping to your routine doesn't cause any harm, it isn't essential for good dental hygiene, according to the American Dental Association. The ADA's fundamental principles of good dental hygiene remain unchanged

Electric Toothbrushes

Electric toothbrushes offer advanced cleaning technology compared to manual toothbrushes, with oscillating or sonic movements that can remove plaque more effectively. Many electric toothbrushes feature built-in timers, pressure sensors, and multiple brushing modes to cater to individual needs and preferences. Some models also connect to smartphone apps to track brushing habits and provide real-time feedback.

The Benefits of Electric Toothbrushes

In today's world, there's a "smart" version of nearly everything, from kitchen appliances to cars. With so many technologically advanced options, it can be challenging to decide which ones are truly beneficial. Electric toothbrushes, invented in 1954 and gaining popularity in the early 2000s, are one such advancement. But do they really make a difference in cleaning your teeth?

Recent studies says that the answer is yes. Electric toothbrushes are generally more effective at removing plaque and keeping teeth clean than manual toothbrushes.

Electric vs. Manual Toothbrush

Studies show that electric toothbrushes outperform manual ones in cleaning teeth, helping prevent cavities and gum disease. Brushing aims to remove plaque and debris, which, if left unchecked, can lead to cavities, tooth decay, gingivitis, and periodontal disease. Plaque can harden into tartar, removable only by a dental professional.

Electric toothbrushes use a rechargeable battery to move a small brush head at high speeds.

Types of Electric Toothbrush Technology:

1. **Oscillating-Rotating Technology:** The brush head spins and rotates to clean. This technology was the first of its kind, with a 2005 study proving it cleans better than manual brushes.
2. **Sonic Technology:** Uses ultrasound and sonic waves to vibrate during brushing. Some models use Bluetooth to send brushing data to a smartphone app, helping you improve your technique over time.

Benefits of Electric Toothbrushes

Using an electric toothbrush can significantly improve oral hygiene and maintain healthy teeth and gums. Patients who struggled with home care showed a decrease in plaque, tartar, and stains when using an electric toothbrush. It's a combination of the brush being more effective and patients brushing longer due to the built-in timers.

Advantages of Electric Toothbrushes:

- **More Reliable Clean:** Electric toothbrushes can produce thousands of strokes per minute, removing plaque more effectively than manual brushing.
- **Specialized Features:** Many models come with timers and pressure sensors to ensure proper brushing duration and pressure. Some have multiple brushing modes for sensitive teeth or gums.
- **Ease of Use:** Electric toothbrushes are easier to use for those with limited dexterity or hand mobility, as they handle most of the brushing work.

Risks of Using an Electric Toothbrush

Like any product, electric toothbrushes have potential downsides. The primary risk is brushing too hard, which can wear down tooth enamel and gums. Brushing harder doesn't equal cleaner teeth; it can damage your enamel and gums,. Pressure sensors on some models can prevent this damage.

Other Considerations:

- **Cost:** Electric toothbrushes are more expensive than manual ones and require regular replacement of brush heads, adding to the cost.
- **Discomfort:** Some people find the sensation of an electric toothbrush uncomfortable, especially those with sensory processing issues.
- **Electricity:** Electric toothbrushes require power, which can be inconvenient without a reliable power source, such as during travel.

Should You Use an Electric Toothbrush?

Electric toothbrushes can enhance your oral hygiene routine, but a manual toothbrush can also be effective when used correctly for the recommended two-minute duration. Always choose a toothbrush with soft or extra-soft bristles and a small brush head to reach behind your molars.

If you're unsure about your brushing technique, ask your dentist, periodontist, or dental hygienist for guidance. They can help you refine your technique to keep plaque and tartar at bay.

Orthodontic Accessories

For individuals with braces or orthodontic appliances, specialized accessories such as floss threaders and orthodontic wax can facilitate oral hygiene and comfort. These products help clean around brackets and wires, prevent irritation, and maintain optimal oral health during orthodontic treatment.

Floss threaders are indispensable tools for maintaining oral hygiene, especially for individuals with braces, bridges, retainers, or other dental appliances that make regular flossing challenging. These flexible, loop-shaped devices help guide dental floss into hard-to-reach areas, ensuring thorough cleaning between teeth and around dental work.

What Are Floss Threaders?

Floss threaders are thin, flexible tools, typically made of nylon or plastic, designed to assist in threading dental floss under braces wires, retainers, bridges, or any other dental appliances. They resemble a large needle with a loop at one end, through which floss is threaded and then guided into tight spaces.

Benefits of Using Floss Threaders

Floss threaders enable effective cleaning between teeth and around dental appliances, reducing the risk of plaque buildup, cavities, and gum disease. They make it easier to reach areas that are typically inaccessible with regular flossing, ensuring a more comprehensive clean. Floss threaders can be used with any type of dental floss, allowing for personalized oral care routines.

By incorporating these advanced oral care techniques and products into a comprehensive oral hygiene routine, individuals can achieve superior plaque control, fresher breath, and healthier gums. Consulting with a dentist or dental hygienist can help determine which advanced oral care strategies are most suitable for individual needs and goals.

11

The Importance of Oral Health

Understanding the Link Between Oral Health and Overall Health

The mouth, often considered the gateway to the body, plays a crucial role in maintaining overall health. Beyond its fundamental functions in eating, speaking, and expressing emotions, oral health has profound implications for systemic well-being. Emerging research continues to unravel the intricate connections between oral health and various systemic conditions, underscoring the importance of comprehensive dental care in promoting overall health.

The oral cavity is a bustling ecosystem, home to billions of bacteria. While many of these microorganisms are harmless and even beneficial, poor oral hygiene can lead to an overgrowth of harmful bacteria. This imbalance can cause periodontal disease, which we already know as a condition that affects the tissues around the teeth. Periodontal disease is not only a leading cause of tooth loss but also a significant contributor to systemic inflammation.

One of the key ways in which oral health is connected to overall health is through inflammation and infection. When you have gum disease or other oral health issues, the inflammation in your mouth can spread to other parts of your body, leading to systemic inflammation. This can contribute to a range of health problems, including heart disease, stroke, and diabetes. By maintaining good oral hygiene and addressing any dental issues promptly, you can help reduce inflammation in your body and protect your overall health.

Understanding the link between oral health and overall health is crucial for individuals who are looking to maintain good health. Many people may not realize that the health of their mouth can have a significant impact on their overall well-being. Poor oral health has been linked to a variety of health conditions, including heart disease, diabetes, and even certain types of cancer. By taking care of your oral health, you can potentially prevent these serious health issues.

Cardiovascular Diseases

Periodontal (gum) disease is associated with a higher risk of cardiovascular diseases such as heart disease, strokes, and atherosclerosis.

Digestive Issues

Poor oral health can affect the ability to chew and properly digest food, leading to gastrointestinal problems

Pregnancy Complications

Periodontal disease has been linked to pregnancy complications such as premature birth and low birth weight babies

Kidney Disease

Individuals with CKD (Chronic kidney disease) are more prone to periodontal disease, and conversely, severe gum disease can worsen kidney function.

The Immune System and Inflammatory Response

The mouth serves as the entry point to both the digestive and respiratory systems, making it a critical barrier against germs. Poor oral hygiene can compromise this barrier, allowing bacteria to enter the bloodstream and trigger systemic inflammation.

Respiratory Problems

Bacterial infections in the mouth can worsen respiratory problems such as bronchitis, pneumonia and emphysema

Diabetes

Your oral health can interfere with your nutrition, increasing the chance of diseases such as diabetes

Mental Health

Pain and discomfort associated with dental problems can have a negative impact on emotional well-being and quality of life.

Neurological Disorders

Chronic periodontal disease and tooth loss have been associated with cognitive decline. The proposed mechanism involves the translocation of oral bacteria to the brain

Emerging research suggests a connection between oral health and neurological conditions, including Alzheimer's disease and other forms of dementia. Furthermore, systemic inflammation from periodontal disease may exacerbate neurodegenerative processes, highlighting the need for further investigation into these connections.

The systemic inflammation caused by periodontal disease can lead to increased levels of C-reactive protein and other inflammatory markers, which are detrimental to kidney health. Moreover, patients with CKD (Chronic kidney disease) often have compromised immune systems, making them more susceptible to oral infections that can further complicate their condition.

Chronic inflammation is a well-established risk factor for numerous diseases, including autoimmune disorders, arthritis, and chronic obstructive pulmonary disease (COPD). For instance, individuals with rheumatoid arthritis are more likely to experience severe periodontal disease, suggesting a reciprocal relationship where inflammation in one system exacerbates the other.

Maintaining good oral hygiene habits can go a long way in preventing costly dental problems and saving you money in the long run. Simple practices like brushing twice a day, flossing daily, and using fluoride toothpaste can help keep your mouth healthy and reduce the need for expensive treatments. Regular dental check-ups and cleanings are also crucial, as they allow your dentist to catch any issues early and provide preventive care.

Oral health's impact on overall health extends beyond the commonly known connections with cardiovascular disease, diabetes, respiratory infections, and pregnancy complications. As research deepens, the multifaceted links between oral health and various systemic conditions become increasingly apparent. This highlights the importance of approaching a health care that incorporates oral health as a fundamental component.

Another important aspect of the link between oral health and overall health is the role of nutrition. A healthy diet is essential for maintaining good oral health, as well as overall health. Foods high in sugar and carbohydrates can contribute to tooth decay and gum disease, while foods rich in vitamins and minerals can help strengthen your teeth and gums. By eating a balanced diet and avoiding sugary and processed foods, you can support your oral health and save money on expensive dental treatments.

12

Nutrition for a Healthy Mouth

The Impact of Diet on Oral Health

How Different Foods Impact Teeth and Gums

Your diet plays a crucial role in maintaining oral health. The types of food and drinks you consume can significantly impact the health of your teeth and gums. Here's a detailed look at how different foods affect your oral health:

Sugary Foods and Drinks

Sugary foods and drinks are one of the leading causes of tooth decay. The bacteria in your mouth feed on sugars and produce acids that attack tooth enamel, leading to cavities. One of the most important aspects of a healthy diet for your oral health is limiting sugary foods and drinks. Sugary snacks and beverages can feed the bacteria in your mouth, leading to the production of acids that can erode tooth enamel and cause cavities. Instead, opt for nutrient-rich foods such as fruits, vegetables, lean proteins, and whole grains. These foods can help strengthen your teeth and gums and reduce your risk of developing dental problems.

- **Examples**: Candies, cakes, cookies, sodas, fruit juices, and sugary cereals.
- **Consequences**: Frequent consumption of these items increases the risk of cavities and other dental problems.

Acidic Foods and Drinks

Acidic foods and drinks can erode tooth enamel over time, making teeth more susceptible to decay and sensitivity.

- **Examples**: Citrus fruits (oranges, lemons, limes), tomatoes, vinegar, and carbonated beverages.
- **Consequences**: Erosion of enamel can lead to increased tooth sensitivity and higher risk of cavities.

Sticky and Starchy Foods

Foods that are sticky or starchy tend to cling to teeth and are harder to clean off. This provides a prolonged food source for bacteria, increasing acid production.

- **Examples**: Caramel, taffy, dried fruits, bread, and potato chips.
- **Consequences**: Extended exposure to these foods can lead to tooth decay.

Dairy Products

Dairy products are beneficial for oral health due to their high calcium and phosphate content, which help to remineralize tooth enamel.

- **Examples**: Milk, cheese, yogurt.
- **Benefits**: Cheese also stimulates saliva production, which helps to neutralize acids in the mouth and wash away food particles.

Fruits and Vegetables

Crunchy fruits and vegetables help clean teeth surfaces and stimulate gums, promoting oral health.

- **Examples**: Apples, carrots, celery, and leafy greens.
- **Benefits**: These foods increase saliva production, which is a natural defense against cavities and gum disease.

Nuts and Seeds

Nuts and seeds are rich in essential nutrients like calcium and phosphates that are important for dental health. Chewing nuts also promotes saliva production.

- **Examples**: Almonds, walnuts, chia seeds, and flaxseeds.
- **Benefits**: They help strengthen teeth and reduce the risk of tooth decay.

Water

Water is essential for maintaining oral health. It helps to wash away food particles and bacteria, reducing the risk of decay. In addition to limiting sugary foods, it is also important to stay hydrated and drink plenty of water throughout the day. Water helps to wash away food particles and bacteria that can lead to plaque buildup and tooth decay. Avoid sugary drinks such as soda and sports drinks, as these can be detrimental to your oral health. Instead, choose water or unsweetened beverages to keep your mouth healthy and hydrated.

- **Benefits**: Drinking water, especially fluoridated water, helps strengthen teeth and prevent cavities. It also helps prevent dry mouth, which can lead to dental problems.

Sugar-Free Gum

Chewing sugar-free gum after meals can help clean teeth and freshen breath. It stimulates saliva production, which neutralizes acids and washes away food particles.

- **Examples**: Gum containing xylitol, a natural sweetener that reduces the risk of cavities.
- **Benefits**: Helps maintain oral hygiene on the go and provides a temporary solution when brushing isn't possible.

Whole Grains

Whole grains provide essential nutrients that support overall health, including oral health. They are less likely to cause spikes in blood sugar, which can affect oral health.

- **Examples**: Brown rice, whole wheat bread, oatmeal, and quinoa.
- **Benefits**: Rich in fiber and other nutrients, whole grains help maintain steady blood sugar levels and promote overall health, including healthy gums

Another important aspect of a healthy diet for your oral health is getting enough calcium and vitamin D. These nutrients are essential for strong teeth and bones, and a deficiency can increase your risk of developing dental issues such as tooth decay and gum disease. Incorporate calcium-rich foods such as dairy products, leafy greens, and almonds into your diet, and consider taking a vitamin D supplement if needed.

Overall, the impact of diet on oral health cannot be overstated. By making smart food choices and prioritizing nutrient-rich foods, you can help maintain a healthy mouth. Remember to limit sugary foods and drinks, stay hydrated with water, and incorporate calcium and vitamin D into your diet to support strong teeth and gums. With a little effort and planning, you can keep your smile bright and your wallet happy.

Budget-Friendly Foods That Promote Oral Health

In fact, there are many budget-friendly foods that can help promote oral health without costing a fortune. By incorporating these foods into your diet, you can improve your oral health while also saving money on expensive dental treatments. In this subchapter, we will explore some of the best budget-friendly foods that promote oral health.

One of the most budget-friendly foods that promote oral health is crunchy fruits and vegetables. Foods like apples, carrots, and celery can help clean your teeth and gums as you chew, reducing the risk of cavities and gum disease. These foods also stimulate saliva production, which helps wash away food particles and bacteria that can lead to oral health issues. Best of all, these fruits and vegetables are often inexpensive and widely available, making them a great option for those on a budget.

Another budget-friendly food that promotes oral health is yogurt. Yogurt is high in calcium and protein, which are essential nutrients for maintaining strong teeth and bones. Additionally, yogurt contains probiotics, which can help balance the bacteria in your mouth and reduce the risk of cavities and gum disease. Opt for plain, unsweetened yogurt to avoid added sugars, which can contribute to tooth decay.

Whole grains are another budget-friendly food that can promote oral health. Foods like brown rice, whole wheat bread, and oatmeal are rich in fiber, which can help scrub away plaque and prevent cavities. Whole grains also contain vitamins and minerals that are important for oral health, such as vitamin B and iron. Additionally, whole grains are often more affordable than processed grains, making them a great choice for those looking to save money on their dental care.

Lastly, lean proteins like chicken, turkey, and fish can also promote oral health without breaking the bank. Protein is essential for repairing and maintaining the tissues in your mouth, including your gums and teeth. Additionally, lean proteins are often more affordable than red meats, making them a great option for those on a budget. By incorporating these budget-friendly foods into your diet, you can improve your oral health without spending a lot of money. Remember, good oral health starts with a healthy diet, so make sure to prioritize these foods in your meals for a healthy mouth.

Recipes and Meal Planning Tips

Incorporating tooth-friendly foods into your diet can be both delicious and economical. Here are some recipes and meal planning tips to help you maintain optimal oral health while sticking to a budget.

10 Breakfast Recipes

By incorporating these budget-friendly breakfast recipes into your routine, you can start your day with nutritious meals that support your oral health. Remember, a balanced breakfast helps maintain strong teeth and gums, providing essential nutrients to keep your mouth healthy

1. Banana Toast

- **Ingredients**:
- 2 slices of whole grain bread
- 2 tablespoons of peanut butter
- 1 banana, sliced

Instructions:

- Toast the bread slices.
- Spread peanut butter on each slice.
- Top with banana slices.
- **Benefits**: Whole grains provide fiber, while peanut butter and bananas offer protein and essential nutrients that help maintain strong teeth and gums.

2. Overnight Oats

- **Ingredients**:
- 1/2 cup rolled oats
- 1/2 cup milk (or a dairy alternative)
- 1/2 cup plain yogurt
- 1 tablespoon chia seeds
- 1/2 cup mixed berries (fresh or frozen)
- 1 teaspoon honey (optional)

Instructions:

- In a jar or container, combine oats, milk, yogurt, chia seeds, and berries.
- Stir well and refrigerate overnight.
- In the morning, stir again and add honey if desired.
- **Benefits**: This easy-to-make breakfast is rich in fiber, calcium, and antioxidants, which support overall oral health.

3. Spinach and Cheese Omelette

- **Ingredients**:
- 2 eggs
- 1/4 cup milk
- 1/2 cup fresh spinach, chopped
- 1/4 cup shredded cheese (cheddar or your choice)
- Salt and pepper to taste

- 1 teaspoon olive oil

Instructions:
- Whisk eggs and milk in a bowl, season with salt and pepper.
- Heat olive oil in a pan over medium heat.
- Add spinach and cook until wilted.
- Pour in the egg mixture and cook until the edges start to set.
- Sprinkle cheese on one half of the omelette, fold the other half over the cheese, and cook until eggs are fully set and cheese is melted.
- **Benefits**: Eggs provide protein and vitamin D, spinach is rich in vitamins and minerals, and cheese offers calcium for strong teeth.

4. Cottage Cheese with Pineapple

- **Ingredients**:
- 1 cup cottage cheese
- 1/2 cup pineapple chunks (fresh or canned, drained)

Instructions:
- Combine cottage cheese and pineapple chunks in a bowl.
- Mix well and serve.
- **Benefits**: Cottage cheese is high in calcium and protein, while pineapple provides vitamin C, promoting healthy gums.

5. Berry Smoothie

- **Ingredients**:
- 1 cup milk (or a dairy alternative)
- 1/2 cup plain yogurt
- 1 cup mixed berries (fresh or frozen)
- 1 tablespoon honey (optional)
- 1 tablespoon ground flaxseed (optional)

Instructions:
- Combine all ingredients in a blender.
- Blend until smooth.
- Pour into a glass and serve.
- **Benefits**: This smoothie is packed with calcium, protein, and antioxidants, supporting overall and oral health.

6. Avocado Toast

- **Ingredients**:
- 1 ripe avocado
- 2 slices whole grain bread
- Salt and pepper to taste
- 1 tablespoon lemon juice (optional)

Instructions:

- Toast the bread slices.
- Mash the avocado in a bowl and season with salt, pepper, and lemon juice if desired.
- Spread the avocado mixture on the toast.
- **Benefits**: Avocado is rich in healthy fats and vitamins, while whole grain bread provides fiber.

7. Greek Yogurt with Granola and Fruit

- **Ingredients**:
- 1 cup plain Greek yogurt
- 1/4 cup granola
- 1/2 cup mixed berries or sliced fruit

Instructions:

- Spoon the Greek yogurt into a bowl.
- Top with granola and fruit.
- **Benefits**: Greek yogurt is high in protein and calcium, granola adds fiber, and fruit provides essential vitamins and antioxidants.

8. Apple Cinnamon Oatmeal

- **Ingredients**:
- 1/2 cup rolled oats
- 1 cup water or milk
- 1 apple, diced
- 1 teaspoon cinnamon
- 1 tablespoon honey or maple syrup (optional)

Instructions:

- Combine oats, water or milk, apple, and cinnamon in a pot.

- Bring to a boil, then reduce heat and simmer until oats are cooked and apple is tender, about 5-7 minutes.
- Stir in honey or maple syrup if desired.
- **Benefits**: Oats are a great source of fiber, and apples provide natural sweetness along with vitamins and minerals.

9. Banana Pancakes

- **Ingredients**:
- 1 ripe banana
- 2 eggs
- 1/4 teaspoon baking powder
- 1/2 teaspoon vanilla extract (optional)
- 1/4 teaspoon cinnamon (optional)
- 1 teaspoon butter or cooking spray for the pan

Instructions:

- Mash the banana in a bowl.
- Whisk in the eggs, baking powder, vanilla extract, and cinnamon.
- Heat a non-stick pan over medium heat and add a small amount of butter or cooking spray.
- Pour batter into the pan to form small pancakes and cook until bubbles form on the surface, then flip and cook until golden brown.
- **Benefits**: These pancakes are naturally sweet and nutritious, with no added sugar. They provide protein from the eggs and potassium from the banana.

10. Smoothie Bowl

- **Ingredients**:
- 1 frozen banana
- 1/2 cup frozen berries
- 1/2 cup plain yogurt
- 1/2 cup milk (or dairy alternative)
- Toppings: granola, fresh fruit, nuts, seeds

Instructions:

- Blend the frozen banana, frozen berries, yogurt, and milk until smooth.
- Pour into a bowl and add your favorite toppings.

- **Benefits**: Smoothie bowls are versatile and can be packed with various nutrients, including protein, fiber, and healthy fats.

10 Lunch Recipes

These lunch recipes are designed to be both nutritious and budget-friendly, supporting your oral health by providing essential vitamins, minerals, and nutrients. Enjoy these delicious meals while maintaining strong teeth and healthy gums.

1. Quinoa and Veggie Salad

- **Ingredients**:
- 1 cup cooked quinoa
- 1/2 cup cherry tomatoes, halved
- 1/2 cucumber, diced
- 1/4 cup red onion, finely chopped
- 1/4 cup feta cheese, crumbled
- 2 tablespoons olive oil
- 1 tablespoon lemon juice
- Salt and pepper to taste

Instructions:

- In a large bowl, combine quinoa, tomatoes, cucumber, red onion, and feta cheese.
- Drizzle with olive oil and lemon juice, then toss to coat.
- Season with salt and pepper.

Benefits: Quinoa is rich in protein and fiber, while vegetables provide essential vitamins and minerals that promote gum health.

2. Chicken and Avocado Wrap

- **Ingredients**:
- 1 whole grain tortilla
- 1/2 cup cooked chicken breast, sliced
- 1/2 avocado, sliced
- 1/4 cup mixed greens
- 1 tablespoon hummus

Instructions:

- Spread hummus on the tortilla.
- Layer chicken, avocado, and mixed greens on top.
- Roll up the tortilla and slice in half.
- **Benefits**: Chicken provides lean protein, while avocado is rich in healthy fats and vitamins that support overall health.

3. Lentil Soup

- **Ingredients**:
- 1 cup lentils, rinsed
- 1 carrot, diced
- 1 celery stalk, diced
- 1 onion, chopped
- 2 garlic cloves, minced
- 1 can diced tomatoes
- 4 cups vegetable broth
- 1 teaspoon cumin
- Salt and pepper to taste
- 1 tablespoon olive oil

Instructions:

- Heat olive oil in a pot over medium heat. Add onion, carrot, celery, and garlic, and cook until softened.
- Add lentils, diced tomatoes, vegetable broth, and cumin.
- Bring to a boil, then reduce heat and simmer for 30 minutes, or until lentils are tender.
- Season with salt and pepper.
- **Benefits**: Lentils are high in protein and fiber, which help maintain healthy gums and teeth.

4. Spinach and Strawberry Salad

- **Ingredients**:
- 2 cups fresh spinach
- 1/2 cup sliced strawberries
- 1/4 cup walnuts, chopped
- 1/4 cup feta cheese, crumbled
- 2 tablespoons balsamic vinaigrette

Instructions:
- In a large bowl, combine spinach, strawberries, walnuts, and feta cheese.
- Drizzle with balsamic vinaigrette and toss to coat.
- **Benefits**: Spinach and strawberries provide antioxidants and vitamins that promote gum health, while walnuts offer healthy fats.

5. Tuna Salad with Greek Yogurt

- **Ingredients**:
- 1 can tuna, drained (you can change the tune for other fish)
- 1/4 cup plain Greek yogurt
- 1 celery stalk, diced
- 1 tablespoon lemon juice
- Salt and pepper to taste
- Whole grain crackers or lettuce leaves for serving

Instructions:
- In a bowl, mix tuna, Greek yogurt, celery, and lemon juice until well combined.
- Season with salt and pepper.
- Serve with whole grain crackers or in lettuce leaves.
- **Benefits**: Greek yogurt provides probiotics and protein, while tuna is a great source of lean protein and omega-3 fatty acids.

6. Chickpea and Veggie Stir-Fry

- **Ingredients**:
- 1 can chickpeas, drained and rinsed
- 1 cup mixed vegetables (such as bell peppers, broccoli, and carrots)
- 2 tablespoons soy sauce
- 1 tablespoon olive oil
- 1 garlic clove, minced
- 1 teaspoon ginger, minced

Instructions:
- Heat olive oil in a pan over medium heat. Add garlic and ginger, and cook until fragrant.
- Add mixed vegetables and cook until tender.
- Stir in chickpeas and soy sauce, and cook for an additional 5 minutes.
- **Benefits**: Chickpeas are high in fiber and protein, and the vegetables provide essential nutrients for gum health.

7. Turkey and Veggie Stuffed Peppers

- **Ingredients**:
- 4 bell peppers, tops cut off and seeds removed
- 1/2 pound ground turkey
- 1 cup cooked brown rice
- 1/2 cup diced tomatoes
- 1/2 onion, chopped
- 1 teaspoon cumin
- 1 teaspoon paprika
- Salt and pepper to taste
- 1 tablespoon olive oil

Instructions:

- Preheat oven to 375°F (190°C).
- Heat olive oil in a pan over medium heat. Add onion and cook until softened.
- Add ground turkey, cumin, paprika, salt, and pepper, and cook until turkey is browned.
- Stir in cooked rice and diced tomatoes.
- Stuff each bell pepper with the turkey mixture and place in a baking dish.
- Bake for 25-30 minutes, or until peppers are tender.
- **Benefits**: Ground turkey provides lean protein, while bell peppers are rich in vitamins A and C, supporting gum health.

8. Egg Salad Lettuce Wraps

- **Ingredients**:
- 4 hard-boiled eggs, chopped
- 1/4 cup plain Greek yogurt
- 1 tablespoon Dijon mustard
- 1 celery stalk, diced
- Salt and pepper to taste
- Lettuce leaves for serving

Instructions:

- In a bowl, mix chopped eggs, Greek yogurt, Dijon mustard, and celery until well combined.
- Season with salt and pepper.
- Serve in lettuce leaves.

- **Benefits**: Eggs provide protein and essential vitamins, while Greek yogurt adds probiotics and creaminess without the fat of mayonnaise.

9. Veggie and Hummus Sandwich

- **Ingredients**:
- 2 slices whole grain bread
- 2 tablespoons hummus
- 1/4 cucumber, sliced
- 1/2 bell pepper, sliced
- 1/4 cup shredded carrots
- 1/4 cup mixed greens

Instructions:

- Spread hummus on each slice of bread.
- Layer cucumber, bell pepper, shredded carrots, and mixed greens on one slice.
- Top with the other slice of bread and cut in half.
- **Benefits**: Hummus provides protein and healthy fats, while the veggies offer a variety of vitamins and minerals.

10. Salmon and Avocado Salad

- **Ingredients**:
- 1 can salmon, drained
- 1 avocado, diced
- 1/4 cup red onion, finely chopped
- 1 tablespoon lemon juice
- Salt and pepper to taste
- Mixed greens for serving

Instructions:

- In a bowl, combine salmon, avocado, red onion, and lemon juice.
- Season with salt and pepper.
- Serve over mixed greens.
- **Benefits**: Salmon provides omega-3 fatty acids and protein, while avocado offers healthy fats and vitamins.

10 Snack Ideas

These snacks are designed to be both nutritious and good for your teeth and gums. By incorporating these healthy options into your diet, you can enjoy delicious snacks while promoting strong teeth and healthy gums.

1. Apple Slices with Almond Butter

- **Ingredients**:
- 1 apple, sliced
- 2 tablespoons almond butter (or any nut butter)

Instructions:

- Slice the apple into wedges.
- Serve with almond butter for dipping.
- **Benefits**: Apples are high in fiber and water, which help clean teeth and stimulate saliva production. Almond butter provides healthy fats and protein.

2. Carrot and Celery Sticks with Hummus

- **Ingredients**:
- 2 carrots, cut into sticks
- 2 celery stalks, cut into sticks
- 1/2 cup hummus

Instructions:

- Arrange carrot and celery sticks on a plate.
- Serve with hummus for dipping.
- **Benefits**: Crunchy vegetables help clean teeth and gums, while hummus provides protein and healthy fats.

3. Cheese and Whole Grain Crackers

- **Ingredients**:
- 1/4 cup cubed cheese (cheddar, mozzarella, or your choice)
- 8-10 whole grain crackers

Instructions:

- Arrange cheese cubes and crackers on a plate.
- **Benefits**: Cheese is rich in calcium and phosphate, which strengthen tooth enamel, and whole grain crackers provide fiber.

4. Greek Yogurt with Berries

- **Ingredients**:
- 1 cup plain Greek yogurt
- 1/2 cup mixed berries (fresh or frozen)

Instructions:

- Top Greek yogurt with mixed berries.
- **Benefits**: Greek yogurt is high in calcium and protein, while berries provide antioxidants and vitamins that promote gum health.

5. Cucumber and Tomato Salad

- **Ingredients**:
- 1 cucumber, sliced
- 1 cup cherry tomatoes, halved
- 1 tablespoon olive oil
- 1 tablespoon vinegar
- Salt and pepper to taste

Instructions:

- Combine cucumber and cherry tomatoes in a bowl.
- Drizzle with olive oil and vinegar.
- Season with salt and pepper, and toss to coat.
- **Benefits**: Cucumbers and tomatoes are high in water and fiber, which help clean teeth and gums.

6. Nut and Seed Mix

- **Ingredients**:
- 1/4 cup almonds
- 1/4 cup walnuts
- 1/4 cup sunflower seeds
- 1/4 cup pumpkin seeds

Instructions:

- Mix all nuts and seeds in a bowl.
- **Benefits**: Nuts and seeds are rich in healthy fats, protein, and minerals like calcium and magnesium, which support oral health.

7. Hard-Boiled Eggs

- **Ingredients**:

- 2 eggs

Instructions:
- Place eggs in a pot and cover with water.
- Bring to a boil, then reduce heat and simmer for 9-12 minutes.
- Remove from heat, cool, peel, and enjoy.
- **Benefits**: Eggs are a great source of protein and vitamin D, which are important for healthy teeth and gums.

8. Pear Slices with Cottage Cheese

- **Ingredients**:
- 1 pear, sliced
- 1/2 cup cottage cheese

Instructions:
- Slice the pear and serve with cottage cheese.
- **Benefits**: Pears help stimulate saliva production and clean teeth, while cottage cheese is rich in calcium and protein.

9. Bell Pepper Strips with Guacamole

- **Ingredients**:
- 1 bell pepper, cut into strips
- 1/2 cup guacamole

Instructions:
- Slice the bell pepper into strips.
- Serve with guacamole for dipping.
- **Benefits**: Bell peppers are high in vitamin C, which supports gum health, and guacamole provides healthy fats and vitamins.

10. Smoothie Popsicles

- **Ingredients**:
- 1 banana
- 1/2 cup spinach
- 1/2 cup Greek yogurt
- 1/2 cup milk (or a dairy alternative)
- 1/2 cup mixed berries
- 1 tablespoon honey (optional)

Instructions:

- Blend all ingredients until smooth.
- Pour into popsicle molds and freeze until solid.
- **Benefits**: These popsicles are packed with nutrients like calcium, vitamins, and antioxidants, which support overall and oral health.

10 Dinner Recipes

These dinner recipes are designed to be nutritious and promote oral health, providing essential nutrients that support strong teeth and healthy gums. Enjoy these meals as part of a balanced diet to maintain your oral health.

1. Baked Salmon with Steamed Vegetables

- **Ingredients**:
- 2 salmon fillets
- 1 lemon
- 2 tablespoons olive oil
- Salt and pepper to taste
- 1 cup broccoli florets
- 1 cup carrot sticks

Instructions:

- Preheat oven to 375°F (190°C).
- Place salmon on a baking sheet, drizzle with olive oil, and season with salt and pepper.
- Squeeze lemon juice over the salmon.
- Bake for 20 minutes or until cooked through.
- Steam broccoli and carrots until tender.
- Serve salmon with steamed vegetables.
- **Tip**: Buy frozen salmon and vegetables to save money without sacrificing nutrition.

2. Quinoa-Stuffed Bell Peppers

- **Ingredients**:

- 4 bell peppers, tops cut off and seeds removed
- 1 cup cooked quinoa
- 1 can black beans, drained and rinsed
- 1 cup corn kernels (fresh or frozen)
- 1/2 cup diced tomatoes
- 1 teaspoon cumin
- Salt and pepper to taste
- 1/4 cup shredded cheese (optional)

Instructions:

- Preheat oven to 375°F (190°C).
- In a bowl, mix cooked quinoa, black beans, corn, diced tomatoes, cumin, salt, and pepper.
- Stuff each bell pepper with the quinoa mixture.
- Place stuffed peppers in a baking dish and cover with foil.
- Bake for 25-30 minutes, or until peppers are tender.
- Optional: sprinkle cheese on top and bake uncovered for an additional 5 minutes.
- **Benefits**: Quinoa and black beans provide protein and fiber, while bell peppers are high in vitamins and antioxidants.

3. Chicken and Vegetable Stir-Fry

- **Ingredients**:
- 2 chicken breasts, sliced
- 2 cups mixed vegetables (such as bell peppers, broccoli, and snap peas)
- 2 tablespoons soy sauce
- 1 tablespoon olive oil
- 1 teaspoon minced garlic
- 1 teaspoon minced ginger

Instructions:

- Heat olive oil in a pan over medium-high heat.
- Add garlic and ginger, and cook until fragrant.
- Add chicken slices and cook until browned and cooked through.
- Add mixed vegetables and soy sauce, and stir-fry until vegetables are tender-crisp.
- **Benefits**: Chicken provides lean protein, and vegetables are rich in fiber and vitamins.

4. Lentil and Spinach Curry

- **Ingredients**:
- 1 cup lentils, rinsed
- 2 cups spinach, chopped
- 1 onion, chopped
- 2 garlic cloves, minced
- 1 can diced tomatoes
- 2 cups vegetable broth
- 1 tablespoon curry powder
- 1 tablespoon olive oil
- Salt and pepper to taste

Instructions:

- Heat olive oil in a pot over medium heat.
- Add onion and garlic, and cook until softened.
- Stir in curry powder and cook for 1 minute.
- Add lentils, diced tomatoes, and vegetable broth.
- Bring to a boil, then reduce heat and simmer for 20-25 minutes, or until lentils are tender.
- Stir in chopped spinach and cook until wilted.
- Season with salt and pepper.
- **Benefits**: Lentils are high in protein and fiber, and spinach provides essential vitamins and minerals for oral health.

5. Grilled Chicken Caesar Salad

- **Ingredients**:
- 2 chicken breasts
- 6 cups romaine lettuce, chopped
- 1/4 cup grated Parmesan cheese
- 1/4 cup croutons
- 2 tablespoons Caesar dressing
- 1 tablespoon olive oil
- Salt and pepper to taste

Instructions:

- Season chicken breasts with salt and pepper.
- Heat olive oil in a grill pan over medium-high heat.
- Grill chicken breasts until cooked through, about 5-7 minutes per side.

- Let chicken rest, then slice.
- In a large bowl, toss romaine lettuce with Caesar dressing.
- Top with grilled chicken slices, Parmesan cheese, and croutons.
- **Benefits**: Chicken provides protein, and romaine lettuce is high in vitamins and minerals.

6. Baked Cod with Lemon and Herbs

- **Ingredients**:
- 2 cod fillets
- 2 tablespoons olive oil
- 1 lemon, sliced
- 2 garlic cloves, minced
- 1 tablespoon fresh parsley, chopped
- Salt and pepper to taste

Instructions:

- Preheat oven to 375°F (190°C).
- Place cod fillets on a baking sheet.
- Drizzle with olive oil, and top with minced garlic, lemon slices, and fresh parsley.
- Season with salt and pepper.
- Bake for 15-20 minutes, or until cod is opaque and flakes easily with a fork.
- **Benefits**: Cod is a good source of lean protein and omega-3 fatty acids, and lemon adds vitamin C.

7. Turkey and Spinach Meatballs

- **Ingredients**:
- 1 pound ground turkey
- 1 cup fresh spinach, chopped
- 1/4 cup grated Parmesan cheese
- 1 egg
- 1/4 cup breadcrumbs
- 2 garlic cloves, minced
- 1 tablespoon Italian seasoning
- Salt and pepper to taste

Instructions:

- Preheat oven to 375°F (190°C).
- In a bowl, combine ground turkey, chopped spinach, Parmesan cheese, egg, breadcrumbs, garlic, Italian seasoning, salt, and pepper.

- Form mixture into meatballs and place on a baking sheet.
- Bake for 20-25 minutes, or until meatballs are cooked through.
- **Benefits**: Turkey is a lean protein source, and spinach provides vitamins and minerals that support gum health.

8. Shrimp and Broccoli Stir-Fry

- **Ingredients**:
- 1 pound shrimp, peeled and deveined
- 2 cups broccoli florets
- 1 red bell pepper, sliced
- 2 tablespoons soy sauce
- 1 tablespoon olive oil
- 1 teaspoon minced garlic
- 1 teaspoon minced ginger

Instructions:

- Heat olive oil in a pan over medium-high heat.
- Add garlic and ginger, and cook until fragrant.
- Add shrimp and cook until pink and opaque.
- Remove shrimp and set aside.
- Add broccoli and bell pepper to the pan, and stir-fry until tender-crisp.
- Return shrimp to the pan and add soy sauce.
- Stir to combine and cook for an additional 2 minutes.
- **Benefits**: Shrimp provides lean protein, and broccoli is rich in fiber, vitamins, and minerals.

9. Veggie-Packed Whole Wheat Pasta

- **Ingredients**:
- 8 ounces whole wheat pasta
- 1 cup cherry tomatoes, halved
- 1 zucchini, diced
- 1 yellow squash, diced
- 2 cups fresh spinach
- 2 tablespoons olive oil
- 1 garlic clove, minced
- Salt and pepper to taste
- Grated Parmesan cheese for serving

Instructions:

- Cook whole wheat pasta according to package instructions.
- Heat olive oil in a large pan over medium heat.
- Add garlic and cook until fragrant.
- Add cherry tomatoes, zucchini, and yellow squash, and cook until tender.
- Stir in fresh spinach and cook until wilted.
- Drain pasta and add to the pan, tossing to combine.
- Season with salt and pepper.
- Serve with grated Parmesan cheese.
- **Benefits**: Whole wheat pasta provides fiber, and the variety of vegetables add vitamins and minerals.

10. Baked Chicken with Sweet Potatoes and Brussels Sprouts

- **Ingredients**:
- 2 chicken breasts
- 2 sweet potatoes, peeled and cubed
- 2 cups Brussels sprouts, halved
- 2 tablespoons olive oil
- 1 teaspoon garlic powder
- 1 teaspoon paprika
- Salt and pepper to taste

Instructions:

- Preheat oven to 400°F (200°C).
- Place chicken breasts, sweet potatoes, and Brussels sprouts on a baking sheet.
- Drizzle with olive oil and season with garlic powder, paprika, salt, and pepper.
- Toss to coat evenly.
- Bake for 25-30 minutes, or until chicken is cooked through and vegetables are tender.
- **Benefits**: Chicken provides lean protein, and sweet potatoes and Brussels sprouts are rich in vitamins and fiber.

10 Dessert Ideas

These dessert recipes are designed to satisfy your sweet tooth while promoting oral health. Incorporate these healthy options into your diet to enjoy delicious treats that support strong teeth and healthy gums.

1. Greek Yogurt Parfait

- **Ingredients**:
- 1 cup plain Greek yogurt
- 1/2 cup mixed berries (blueberries, strawberries, raspberries)
- 1 tablespoon honey (optional)
- 2 tablespoons granola (preferably low-sugar)

Instructions:

- Layer Greek yogurt, mixed berries, and granola in a glass.
- Drizzle with honey if desired.
- **Benefits**: Greek yogurt is high in calcium and probiotics, and berries are rich in antioxidants.

2. Apple Slices with Cinnamon and Nuts

- **Ingredients**:
- 1 apple, sliced
- 1 teaspoon cinnamon
- 2 tablespoons chopped nuts (almonds, walnuts, pecans)

Instructions:

- Arrange apple slices on a plate.
- Sprinkle with cinnamon and chopped nuts.
- **Benefits**: Apples help clean teeth, and nuts provide healthy fats and protein.

3. Chia Seed Pudding

- **Ingredients**:
- 1/4 cup chia seeds
- 1 cup almond milk (or milk of your choice)
- 1 tablespoon honey or maple syrup

- 1/2 teaspoon vanilla extract
- Fresh fruit for topping (optional)

Instructions:

- Mix chia seeds, almond milk, honey, and vanilla extract in a bowl.
- Cover and refrigerate for at least 4 hours or overnight, until thickened.
- Top with fresh fruit before serving.
- **Benefits**: Chia seeds are rich in fiber and omega-3 fatty acids, which support overall health.

4. Frozen Banana Bites

- **Ingredients**:
- 2 bananas, sliced
- 1/2 cup dark chocolate chips
- 1 tablespoon coconut oil

Instructions:

- Line a baking sheet with parchment paper.
- Melt dark chocolate chips and coconut oil in a microwave-safe bowl, stirring every 30 seconds until smooth.
- Dip banana slices into melted chocolate and place on the baking sheet.
- Freeze for at least 1 hour before serving.
- **Benefits**: Bananas are high in vitamins and minerals, and dark chocolate contains antioxidants.

5. Baked Pears with Honey and Cinnamon

- **Ingredients**:
- 2 pears, halved and cored
- 2 tablespoons honey
- 1 teaspoon cinnamon
- 1/4 cup chopped walnuts

Instructions:

- Preheat oven to 350°F (175°C).
- Place pear halves in a baking dish.
- Drizzle with honey and sprinkle with cinnamon and chopped walnuts.
- Bake for 20-25 minutes, or until pears are tender.
- **Benefits**: Pears help clean teeth, and walnuts provide healthy fats and protein.

6. Cottage Cheese with Pineapple

- **Ingredients**:
- 1 cup cottage cheese
- 1/2 cup fresh pineapple chunks

Instructions:

- Mix cottage cheese and pineapple chunks in a bowl.
- **Benefits**: Cottage cheese is high in calcium and protein, and pineapple contains vitamins and enzymes that promote gum health.

7. Oatmeal Cookies (Low-Sugar)

- **Ingredients**:
- 1 cup rolled oats
- 1/2 cup whole wheat flour
- 1/4 cup unsweetened applesauce
- 1/4 cup honey
- 1 egg
- 1/2 teaspoon baking soda
- 1 teaspoon cinnamon
- 1/2 cup raisins or dark chocolate chips (optional)

Instructions:

- Preheat oven to 350°F (175°C).
- In a bowl, mix rolled oats, whole wheat flour, applesauce, honey, egg, baking soda, and cinnamon until combined.
- Fold in raisins or dark chocolate chips if desired.
- Drop spoonfuls of dough onto a baking sheet.
- Bake for 10-12 minutes, or until edges are golden brown.
- **Benefits**: Oats provide fiber, and using applesauce and honey as sweeteners keeps the sugar content low.

8. Avocado Chocolate Mousse

- **Ingredients**:
- 2 ripe avocados
- 1/4 cup cocoa powder
- 1/4 cup honey or maple syrup
- 1/4 cup almond milk
- 1 teaspoon vanilla extract

Instructions:

- Blend all ingredients in a food processor until smooth and creamy.
- Chill in the refrigerator for at least 1 hour before serving.
- **Benefits**: Avocados provide healthy fats and vitamins, and cocoa powder contains antioxidants.

9. Mango Sorbet

- **Ingredients**:
- 2 ripe mangoes, peeled and chopped
- 1 tablespoon lime juice
- 1 tablespoon honey (optional)
- **Instructions**:
- Blend mangoes, lime juice, and honey in a blender until smooth.
- Pour mixture into a freezer-safe container and freeze for at least 4 hours, stirring every hour to prevent ice crystals.
- **Benefits**: Mangoes are high in vitamins A and C, supporting gum health.

10. Berry and Spinach Smoothie

- **Ingredients**:
- 1 cup mixed berries (fresh or frozen)
- 1 cup fresh spinach
- 1 banana
- 1 cup almond milk (or milk of your choice)
- 1 tablespoon honey (optional)

Instructions:

- Blend all ingredients until smooth.
- Serve immediately.
- **Benefits**: Berries and spinach provide antioxidants and vitamins, and the smoothie is high in fiber.

9. Cheese and Fruit Platter

- **Ingredients**:
- Assorted cheeses (cheddar, mozzarella, etc.)
- Grapes
- Apple slices

- Pear slices

Instructions:

- Arrange cheese and fruit on a platter for a simple, tooth-friendly dessert.
- **Tip**: Look for sales on cheese and buy fruits in season to keep costs low.

10. Yogurt with Honey and Nuts

- **Ingredients**:
- 1 cup plain yogurt
- 1 tablespoon honey
- 2 tablespoons chopped nuts (walnuts, almonds, etc.)

Instructions:

- Top yogurt with honey and chopped nuts.
- **Tip**: Use plain yogurt to avoid added sugars and enjoy the natural sweetness of honey and nuts.

Meal Planning Tips

1. **Plan Ahead**: Create a weekly meal plan to avoid impulse buys and reduce food waste. Use a shopping list based on your meal plan to stay within your budget.
2. **Buy in Bulk**: Purchase non-perishable items like nuts, grains, and canned goods in bulk to save money over time.
3. **Seasonal Shopping**: Choose fruits and vegetables that are in season for the best prices and quality. Farmers' markets and local grocery stores often offer discounts on seasonal produce.
4. **Cook in Batches**: Prepare large batches of meals and portion them out for the week. This saves time and ensures you have healthy meals ready to go.
5. **Use Leftovers**: Incorporate leftovers into new meals. For example, leftover chicken can be used in salads, wraps, or stir-fries.

By incorporating these recipes and meal planning tips into your routine, you can maintain excellent oral health without breaking the bank. Remember, a balanced diet not only supports your overall health but also plays a crucial role in keeping your teeth and gums healthy.

13

How to set up my preventive care strategy?

Developing a personalized preventive care strategy is key to maintaining a healthy mouth and saving money on dental expenses. Start by evaluating your current oral hygiene habits and identifying areas for improvement, commit to brushing and flossing regularly, and consider incorporating additional fluoride products into your routine. Schedule regular dental check-ups and cleanings, and be proactive about addressing any issues that arise. Remember, the key to success is consistency and making oral health a priority in your daily life.

Step One: Me in the mirror

Let's start small, the first step in assessing your oral hygiene and health, look in the mirror to see if you notice any stains, decay or inflammation. If you find any issues with your oral health, make an urgent appointment with your dentist. After evaluating your overall oral health and checking if your hygiene is adequate, it's time for us to implement our BFF routine.

Step Two: Implementing BFF Routine

1. **Set a Regular Time:** Choose a convenient time in your daily routine to brush and floss your teeth. It could be after breakfast and before bed, for example. Consistency is key!
2. **Create a Reward System:** Make brushing and flossing more enjoyable by implementing a reward system. For example, you could treat yourself to a small reward (like a sticker, a favorite snack, or extra screen time) each time you complete your routine for a certain number of days in a row.
3. **Make it Fun:** Turn brushing and flossing into a fun activity! Play your favorite song while you brush, challenge yourself to brush for the duration of a catchy tune, or try brushing and flossing games to make it more enjoyable.
4. **Use Visual Reminders:** Place visual reminders in your bathroom to prompt you to brush and floss. This could be a sticky note on the mirror, a checklist on the wall, or a colorful chart to track your progress.

5. **Set Realistic Goals:** Start with achievable goals, such as brushing and flossing once a day, and gradually increase the frequency or duration as you build the habit.
6. **Celebrate Milestones:** Celebrate your achievements along the way! Whether it's reaching a certain number of consecutive days of brushing and flossing or noticing improvements in your oral health, take a moment to acknowledge your progress and pat yourself on the back.

Note if you have children, you can also establish a the BFF routine with them. The earlier we start getting used to taking care of our oral health, the easier and fewer problems we'll have along the way.

Step Three: Schedule an appointment

To maintain optimal oral health make sure to book regular dental appointments, it will cost you less than a complex treatment. Dental professionals can provide valuable advice, thorough cleanings, and identify any potential issues early on. By keeping up with regular appointments, you can stay on top of your oral hygiene and prevent more serious dental problems in the future.

Step Four: Create a Habit

Consistency is the key to turning a habit into a lifestyle . Incorporate oral hygiene into your daily routine by setting aside time each day specifically for brushing and flossing. Make it a priority, just like eating or sleeping, and stick to it even on busy or stressful days. Remember, a little effort every day goes a long way in maintaining a healthy smile.

Tips for Busy lifestyles

In today's fast-paced world, it can be challenging to prioritize our oral health amidst the demands of work, family, and social commitments. However, neglecting our oral health can have serious consequences, including tooth decay, gum disease, and even more serious health issues such as heart disease and diabetes. With a few simple oral health tips for busy lifestyles, we can ensure that our smiles stay healthy and bright even when life gets hectic.

One of the most important oral health tips for busy lifestyles is to establish a regular oral hygiene routine and stick to it. This means brushing your teeth at least three times a day for two minutes each time, using a fluoride toothpaste and a soft-bristled toothbrush. It's also important to floss at least once a day to remove plaque and food particles from between your teeth. If you find it difficult to find time to brush and floss, try keeping a toothbrush and floss in your purse or car so you can take care of your oral hygiene on the go.

In addition to regular brushing and flossing, it's important to visit your dentist for regular check-ups and cleanings. Ideally, you should see your dentist every six months for a professional cleaning and exam. This will help prevent cavities, gum disease, and other oral health issues before they become serious problems. If you have a busy schedule, try to schedule your dental appointments well in advance and mark them on your calendar so you don't forget.

Another important oral health tip for busy lifestyles is to watch what you eat and drink. Sugary and acidic foods and beverages can contribute to tooth decay and gum disease, so it's important to limit your consumption of these items. Instead, try to eat a balanced diet rich in fruits, vegetables, whole grains, and lean proteins. Drinking plenty of water throughout the day can also help wash away bacteria and food particles that can cause cavities and bad breath.

If you find yourself constantly on the go, it can be tempting to skip brushing and flossing or reach for sugary snacks and drinks for a quick energy boost. However, these habits can have a negative impact on your oral health. Instead, try to plan ahead and pack healthy snacks like fruits, vegetables, nuts, and cheese to have on hand when you're busy. You can also keep a travel-sized toothbrush and toothpaste in your bag so you can freshen up after meals or snacks.

Finally, it's important to protect your teeth and gums from injury during your busy lifestyle. If you participate in sports or activities that could put your mouth at risk, such as contact sports or biking, be sure to wear a mouthguard to prevent injuries. If you grind your teeth at night or during times of stress, talk to your dentist about getting a custom-fitted night guard to protect your teeth from damage.

Information is gold

Staying informed and engaged is crucial to maintaining optimal oral health. This involves keeping up with the latest recommendations for preventive care and actively participating in your oral health management. Here's how you can stay informed and engaged to ensure your preventive care plan is as effective as possible:

The field of dental care is constantly evolving, with new research and technologies emerging regularly. Staying updated on the latest recommendations for preventive care can help you adopt the best practices for your oral health. Subscribe to newsletters from reputable dental organizations, follow dental care experts on social media, and read articles from trusted sources to keep abreast of new developments. Your dentist can also provide you with the latest guidelines during your regular check-ups.

Taking an active role in your oral health means more than just brushing and flossing regularly. Engage with your preventive care plan by setting and tracking your oral health goals. Use tools like dental care apps to monitor your habits and progress. Being proactive helps you stay committed to maintaining good oral hygiene and allows you to notice any changes or issues early on.

Never hesitate to ask your dentist or dental hygienist questions. Whether you're curious about the best techniques for brushing and flossing, or you need clarification on a treatment recommendation, your dental care team is there to help. By asking questions, you ensure that you fully understand your care plan and the reasons behind each recommendation. This understanding empowers you to make informed decisions about your oral health. Your dentist and dental hygienist are your partners in maintaining oral health. Build a strong relationship with them by communicating openly about your health history, any concerns you have, and your goals for your oral health. A good relationship with your care team can make your visits more comfortable and productive, and ensure that you receive personalized care.

Regular dental screenings and exams are vital components of preventive care. These visits allow your dentist to detect potential issues early, when they are most treatable and before they become costly problems. Follow through with the recommended schedule for cleanings, exams, and any necessary screenings, such as X-rays. Staying diligent with these appointments ensures that you maintain optimal oral health.

Take the time to educate yourself about oral health. Read books, attend webinars, and join online forums to learn from experts and fellow patients. Understanding the causes and prevention of common dental issues, such as cavities and gum disease, can motivate you to maintain good habits and seek timely treatment when needed.

Leverage technology to stay on top of your oral health. Use reminder apps to schedule brushing and flossing, track your dental appointments, and monitor your dietary habits. Some apps also provide educational content and tips for improving your oral hygiene practices.

In conclusion, maintaining good oral health is essential for overall well-being, even when life gets busy. By following these simple oral health tips for busy lifestyles, you can ensure that your smile stays healthy and bright for years to come. Remember to brush and floss regularly, visit your dentist for check-ups and cleanings, watch what you eat and drink, and protect your teeth from injury. With a little effort and planning, you can enjoy a healthy smile no matter how busy your life may be.

14

Investing in your oral health, investing in your future

Throughout this book, we have examined the vital relationship between oral health and financial well-being. The insights provided in each chapter serve as a comprehensive guide to understanding the importance of maintaining good oral hygiene and its far-reaching implications.

We explored how dental care expenses can quickly accumulate, emphasizing the necessity of preventive measures to avoid costly treatments. By understanding the financial ramifications of neglecting oral health, you can appreciate the value of investing in regular dental care and hygiene practices.

Learn about the groundwork for recognizing what constitutes good oral hygiene. we highlighted essential practices like proper brushing, flossing, and regular dental check-ups, which are critical for preventing oral diseases and maintaining overall health.

Understanding the Anatomy of your mouth, including the structure and function of your teeth and gums, is crucial for recognizing potential issues early on. This knowledge empowers you to take proactive steps in caring for your oral health and seeking timely professional advice when needed.

We delved into common Issues, where we examined typical problems such as cavities, gum disease, and tooth loss. Each condition was discussed in terms of its impact on health and finances, demonstrating how early intervention and preventive care can significantly reduce long-term costs and improve quality of life.

We underscored the importance of understanding your dental care options and making choices that align with both your health needs and financial situation. By being well-informed, you can navigate the complexities of dental treatments and insurance plans with confidence and clarity.

Highlighted the unique dental care needs at various phases of life—from infancy and childhood through adulthood and into the senior years. Recognizing and addressing these specific needs ensures that your oral care routine is always appropriate and effective.

We debunked common misconceptions, providing you with accurate information to dispel myths that could otherwise hinder your oral hygiene practices. Knowledge is power, and understanding the truth about oral health empowers you to maintain better habits and make smarter decisions.

Offered you practical tips for maintaining excellent oral hygiene without overspending. From cost-effective products to home remedies and preventive strategies, this chapter demonstrated that you don't need to break the bank to achieve and maintain good oral health.

We focused on the foundational elements of oral care, such as proper brushing and flossing techniques. Consistently applying these basics is critical for preventing dental issues and maintaining overall oral health.

Underscored how oral hygiene is integral to overall health. Good oral health can prevent systemic issues, boost self-confidence, and contribute to a higher quality of life. Moreover, recognizing the connection between oral health and overall health underscores the importance of investing in your oral health. By making oral health a priority and embracing its impact on both your oral health and overall health, you are taking control of your dental care and setting yourself up for a healthier and more financially secure future. Your mouth and your wallet will thank you in the long run.

Highlighted the role of diet in maintaining strong teeth and healthy gums. Making informed dietary choices can significantly enhance your oral health, showcasing the connection between what you eat and your dental well-being.

Finally, weprovided a roadmap for developing a personalized preventive care plan. By setting up regular check-ups, adopting consistent oral hygiene habits, and staying vigilant about changes in your oral health, you can prevent problems before they start and save on costly treatments down the line.

Beyond the physical and financial benefits, investing in your oral health can also improve your self-confidence and overall well-being. A healthy smile can boost your self-esteem and make you feel more confident in social and professional settings. It can also improve your relationships with others as a bright smile is often seen as a sign of good health and hygiene. By taking care of your oral health, you are investing in yourself and your future success.

This book has taken you on a comprehensive journey through the multifaceted world of oral health, emphasizing the profound impact that informed decisions and proactive care can have on your well-being and finances. Let's revisit the crucial insights and practical advice offered in each chapter to reinforce the path toward maintaining a healthy mouth and a healthy wallet.

In conclusion, investing in your oral health is essential for maintaining good overall health and well-being. By establishing a good oral hygiene routine, making smart dietary choices, seeking professional dental care when needed, and maintaining regular dental check-ups, you can prevent oral diseases and ensure that your teeth and gums are in good condition. Investing in your oral health can have a lasting impact on your future by reducing the risk of developing serious health conditions, saving you money on costly dental procedures, and improving your self-esteem and confidence. So, take the time to invest in your oral health today for a healthier and brighter future.

Healthy Mouth
Maintain good oral hygiene for a beautiful, confident smile.

Healthy Wallet
Save money by preventing costly dental problems.

Healthy Future
Invest in your oral health to safeguard your overall well-being.

About the Autor

Leonardo Melo is a dentist residing in Brazil, graduated from the Dentistry College of Pernambuco and specialized in dental implants and Oral Health care. He believes that knowledge about the key points of oral health can bring greater longevity to a person's life and, most importantly, enable them to acquire excellent self-esteem and well-being. He said that he will keep working to ensure that information reaches more and more people so that we can achieve a great oral health, well-being and be able to appreciate life the way it should be enjoyed.

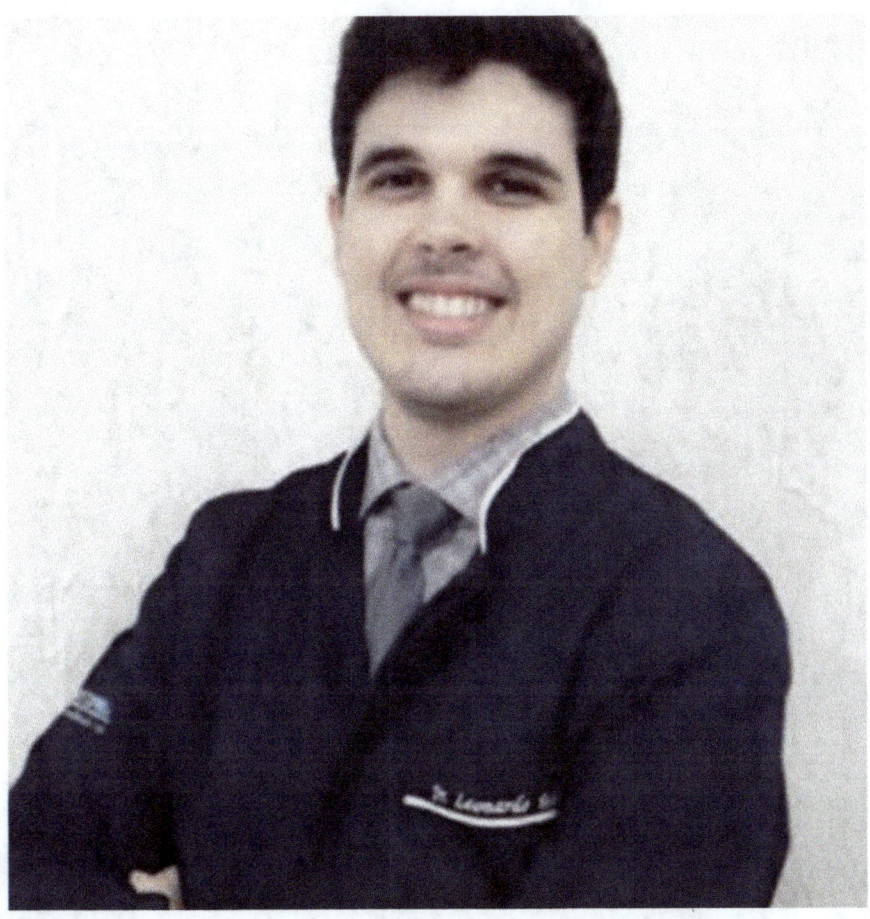

www.ingramcontent.com/pod-product-compliance
Lightning Source LLC
Chambersburg PA
CBHW071518220526
45472CB00003B/1065